Callum's Cure

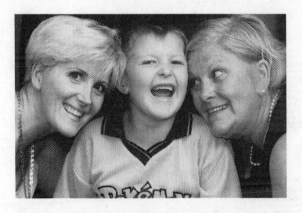

*Happy birthday magic – three generations
born 29 July: Shelley, Callum and Paulina.*

Callum's Cure

A TRIUMPH OF POSITIVE PARENTING

To Claire & all at Yorkshire TV love & best wishes [signature] & Rory x

SHELLEY SYKES

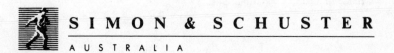

SIMON & SCHUSTER

AUSTRALIA

The advice given in this book is based on the author's experience. Professionals should be consulted for individuals' problems. The author and publisher shall not be responsible for any person with regard to any loss or damage caused directly or indirectly by the information in this book.

First published in Australia in 2003 by
Simon & Schuster (Australia) Pty Limited
20 Barcoo Street, East Roseville NSW 2069

A Viacom Company
Sydney New York London Toronto Singapore

Visit our website at www.simonsaysaustralia.com.au

National Library of Australia
Cataloguing-in-Publication data

Sykes, Shelley
Callum's cure.

Bibliography.
Includes index.
ISBN 0 7318 1200 X

Sykes, Callum – Health. 2. Sykes, Shelley. 3. Cerebral palsied children – Care. 4. Cerebral palsied children – Australia – Biography. 5. Parents of children with Disabilities – Australia – Biography. I. Title.

362.1968360092

Poems by Sylvia G. Poore and Natalie Simon appear with kind permission of the authors.
Cover design by Jason van Genderen, Treehouse Creative
Internal design by Anna Soo
Typesetting by Peter Guo, Letter Spaced
Typeset in Caslon 224 Book 10.5 pt on 15 pt
Printed in Australia by Griffin Press

10 9 8 7 6 5 4 3 2 1

This book is dedicated to my very loving and successful son, Callum Rory, without whom I would not have become the person I am today. May all his wishes and dreams continue to come true.

Contents

Foreword

Raising any child is a challenge for a parent or carer. Raising a child who falls ill adds to that responsibility, but bringing up a child with ongoing health problems brings a whole new meaning to parenting challenges.

There are so many courageous families looking after children with special needs who battle on in silence. *Callum's Cure* describes one family's struggle, from a personal perspective rather than a medical one, and their triumph in raising a happy, positive child, despite the fact that he was born with cerebral palsy.

Shelley and Callum's story highlights real-life issues facing parents raising a child, no matter what their circumstances. Parents and carers can make an enormous difference to the self-esteem and confidence of their children, whether those children are healthy or not. Many parents who learn that their child has a disability do not know where to turn for support and advice. Who better to offer guidance to parents in this situation than a mother who has overcome many daunting obstacles to enable her son to lead a normal life? Shelley has done a wonderful job with Callum Rory.

Callum's Cure has certainly opened my eyes to the issues facing any family raising a child with special needs, perhaps making me more sensitive to the way I relate to my patients and their parents.

As a doctor and surgeon, it is my passion to help children achieve their greatest physical potential. But it is a team effort, and doctors rely heavily on parents to maintain their child's physiotherapy program at home and boost their child's self-esteem.

I believe that Callum's success will inspire many parents to continue to strive for their goals and encourage their children to reach their potential.

Dr Michael R.G. Stenning MBBS, FRACS
Orthopaedic Surgeon
Specialist in Paediatric Orthopaedics
Sydney Children's Hospital, Randwick

Acknowledgments

I would particularly like to thank Andrew Matthews, author of *Follow your Heart*, whose book inspired me to write my own book and to follow my dreams. A special thanks to Anthony Robbins, author of *Unleash the Power Within*, who inspired Callum Rory and I to step up and unleash our power.

Gratitude also to the staff of the Child Development Centre, Airedale Hospital, for their continued emotional and physical support throughout Callum Rory's life. Special thanks to Dr Kate Ward (Children's Paediatric Doctor), Steven Brown and Ruth McAlister (Physiotherapist, now retired), and Judith Holt (Physiotherapist in Sydney).

Heartfelt thanks to Callum Rory's surgeons, Mr Bradbury, Mr Bell and Dr Michael Stenning, who performed Callum's eye and leg operations respectively, and to the nurses who cared for him.

Thanks also to Simon & Schuster, who had the heart and sensitivity to publish this book.

Callum Rory would like to thank his mother and his favourite support teacher, Rachel Dennison.

Introduction

Whatever you can conceive
and dream, you can achieve.

I NOW KNOW that the secret for great parenting is to build our children's confidence, to love unconditionally and to raise their self-esteem. When we do these things, miracles can happen. Hopefully the stories and experiences in this book will give you ideas about how to be a great parent to your own children.

When I first became a parent, I realised that few of us are trained for this most challenging and important of tasks. We are blessed with an immense power to mould and develop the nature and behavioural patterns of our children, building their self-esteem and confidence for the future. Yet most of the time we don't know what we're doing. Our child is like a white canvas waiting for the artist's brush.

Let's face it, we all aim to be happy, healthy and loved, and for our children to be equally happy. So if our goals are so simple, there should be a simple strategy to achieve them. When I was searching for guidance in the best way to raise Callum, I ploughed through hundreds of self-help books and biographies of successful people who had all started out as ordinary, not necessarily clever or advantaged, people. The title of the Australian property magnate John McGrath's book, *You Don't Have To Be Born Brilliant*, is so apt. Through my intuition, my study of counselling, psychology, neuro-linguistic programming (NLP), aromatherapy, reiki, and of course trial and error, I came to the simple conclusion that anyone can learn the skills needed to achieve a goal if they are passionate about it – and most of us *are* passionate about our children. Importantly, in raising our children, we can remain true to who *we* are.

I dream therefore I am ...

All any child wants is to be listened to and loved for who they are, no matter what their circumstances. I realised that all we need to learn as adults is how to raise self-esteem, develop confidence and love unconditionally, since most of us have not been shown how to love without conditions being applied by our own parents or peers. Nor have we been taught how to be great parents.

It is an amazing experience to be able to listen, give love, confidence and self-esteem to our children, as it changes our lives and theirs in the process.

This book has been lovingly written after achieving the unthinkable for my son, Callum Rory, who was born blind with cerebral palsy, but who now can see, walk and is a confident, delightful, happy, normal, cheeky boy. I learnt how to be a great parent to a special-needs child. I want to share my experiences with as many people as possible, so my second baby, this book, was born!

I hope you will be inspired by our story to make a positive difference to your children. If I, as a 'non-mumsy' type, can raise a happy, confident child with the additional challenges of overcoming his medical problems and being a single parent, then I know you can achieve great success with your own family.

Callum's Cure, as I've called it, is the story of our journey together. I was told that Callum Rory may never walk, due to brain damage caused by a car accident when I was pregnant. Cerebral palsy cannot be 'cured', but huge strides can be made towards achieving a 'normal' life. Callum at 11 years old says, 'The past doesn't equal the future. It isn't what happens to you in life that matters, it's what you do about it that counts.' With a brilliant smile, sparkly eyes that can see without the aid of glasses, and the longest legs in his class, Callum Rory is a miracle on walking legs.

If I can achieve miracles, as a sole parent raising a boy with health problems, then so can you. We can't follow in anyone else's footsteps, but we can learn valuable lessons from each other. It is never too late. The past does not equal the future!

You may find some parts of this book challenging, depending on what stage you have reached with your children and other relationships at this time.

I trust that *Callum's Cure* will give you insight into how your family can thrive amidst the challenges by:

- showing how to create a fun family atmosphere
- providing tips and ideas for dealing with guilt
- demonstrating how to show compassion, not just to others but to ourselves
- showing how to understand and accept others' inability to cope with difficult situations
- revealing the pain a child feels in rejection and how you can overcome their insecurities, and
- highlighting the importance of surrounding yourself with true friends to help you through the tough times.

You will see that it hasn't all been smooth sailing for us. There have been many setbacks on our journey, but Callum's story demonstrates that it is possible to overcome the hurdles that life puts in your way, and that there is always a silver lining – miracles do happen. I hope that reading about our experiences will lighten your load, giving you the knowledge and confidence to venture to more exciting and rewarding levels.

I also hope that *Callum's Cure* gives you the confidence to become the great parent or carer you were always meant to be, confirms that you are already on track, and reaffirms your commitment to your children and to your dreams. May reading our story help you to live with courage, passion and faith.

A boy called Callum

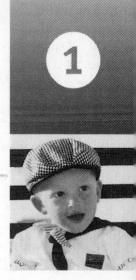

Nothing can resist the human will
that will stake even its existence
on its stated purpose.

Benjamin Disraeli

DO YOU REMEMBER how you felt when you first learnt that you were pregnant or were going to be a dad? The feeling for most people is a combination of amazement, excitement, fear and, above all, pure joy. Relief, too, that you have begun the process of fulfilling the basic human need to reproduce. Mission two accomplished, mission one having been the search for a mate.

In 1991, while on holiday in South Africa visiting friends I had made when I lived there in the 1980s, I began to feel unwell. Bilharzia and malaria are prevalent in Africa, and I had just been waterskiing in possibly infected water. I didn't fancy returning to the United

Kingdom with a dreaded disease the English doctors may not be able to identify!

Several years earlier I had been infected with spinal and cerebral meningitis after swallowing infected water in the Knysna River, which had me close to death in intensive care for several weeks. The South African health system was second to none, leading the world in medical research into heart transplants, test-tube babies and rare diseases. Thanks to new drugs and the advanced medical techniques of the South African doctors caring for me, I recovered. I was so very lucky.

As a healthy and energetic person with above-average fitness, and with memories of my earlier experiences in South Africa, I panicked and booked myself into a clinic in Johannesburg, convinced that I had caught something nasty. I didn't want to take any chances with my health. My husband Leigh and I were utterly shocked but thrilled to learn that I was suffering from nothing more serious than morning sickness!

My sympathies go out to anyone suffering this side effect of pregnancy. Before experiencing it for myself, I had no idea what it was like. I thought that pregnant women were just playing on the sympathy vote. But it's like having really bad seasickness morning, noon and night. Disgusting and terribly draining – death almost felt like a preferable option, at times!

At Sandton Clinic in Johannesburg I was told that I was expecting a baby boy. I was even shown his little heartbeat on a computer screen. It was amazing to see, as he was only a few weeks gestated. Back home in England, our families were overjoyed to hear that we would soon be parents.

Parents – and me a mother ... wow, that sounded so grown up! Mind you, I was only 29 years young. After the initial elation, reality started to hit home ... I was scared. We had decided to try for a family two years earlier, but it was apparent that I couldn't conceive. I didn't have periods, which my doctor assumed was an effect of the contraceptive I was on that was administered by injection every three months. It was expected that my periods would return once the injections were stopped, but it could take time for my body to readjust. Two years was excessive, and though I was somewhat disappointed at the time, I focused on all the wonderful things in our lives. We had a busy schedule and we crammed a lot into our days. We had a beautiful home and future plans to live abroad.

I had decided to put my energies into creating my dream career. By this time I was a successful business-woman, entrepreneur, director of my own companies, and I was working my way up the ranks in television and the media. I was loving every minute of it. My husband worked away a lot on IT projects from Mondays to Fridays, giving me the freedom to develop my career and to socialise.

Being apart most of the week, we spent our weekends in bed or enjoyed romantic weekends in Europe. It was a wonderful lifestyle. So was I really ready for motherhood? I still hadn't learnt how to cook! And the thought of stinky nappies ... yuck! I couldn't envisage myself pushing a pram around in high heels! Then there was childbirth to consider: it was sure to hurt. Why oh why hadn't they developed the instant test-tube baby yet? I had come to realise that babies are not always like the cute three- to six-month-olds depicted in advertising.

Teeny, weeny babies are so fragile and so ugly, I thought. My sister Nichola had had a cute little baby girl, Amber, who I loved dressing up in beautiful little outfits. But the idea of holding her when she was a newborn was too scary. I liked babies when they could talk and laugh, and when you could give them back to their parents.

However, when the time came for me to have my first ultrasound scan at 13 weeks pregnant, at Airedale Hospital, Yorkshire, the realisation that a baby was indeed developing inside me was both exciting and sobering. I began talking to the foetus every day, and I scoured all the baby stores, oohing and aahing over the tiny clothes and all the accessories that were available. I was a typical first-time mum to be. I set up a beautiful nursery stacked with the full range of cuddly Beatrix Potter characters for our baby, and bought little velour romper suits in preparation for the birth. My girlfriends just adored the impractical designer baby room I had created. The baby

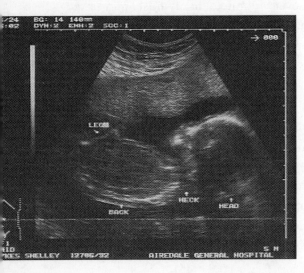

Ultrasound scan of baby Sykes. Life's creation – my baby.

shower was just as exciting to my girlfriends as my hens' party had been!

My very special friend Sonya, who lived in Holland, had not been able to fly to England for the baby shower. Instead I planned a quiet, relaxing five-day holiday with Sonya and her family in Holland at 32 weeks pregnant. It was a weird time for me, because the baby had begun to do somersaults in my stomach and I could often see his little legs or arms pushing against my bloated tummy like some alien from a sci-fi movie. I imagined that the trip to Holland would be my last girlie holiday for a while, and I wasn't wrong …

Sonya and I were involved in a serious car accident. A Mercedes suddenly pulled out onto the highway in front of us, colliding with our vehicle. Sonya suffered severe shock and a broken tooth. Her car was written off. I suffered a broken sternum, my stomach was bruised black and blue, I had cuts to my leg, and severe whiplash. Our relaxing, laughter-filled holiday had come to an abrupt end.

In the ensuing days and weeks I was petrified that the baby had died inside of me, because it had stopped moving since the accident.

In the hospital, the doctors confirmed the baby's little heartbeat, but the following weeks were very stressful. Outwardly I put on a smiling face, but I was terribly anxious. My instincts were telling me that something just wasn't right with my unborn baby. My husband thought that I was worrying unnecessarily, so I buried my concerns inside.

My husband was unable to attend any of the antenatal classes after our initial hospital visit, because he was still working away from home. Fortunately for me, my new friends Emma and Richard accompanied me to all the classes. It was a joke that Richard had two pregnant women, one on each arm. He was so excited about his and Emma's forthcoming first child. He would pant and breathe with the two of us, and would revive me after my occasional fainting spells during the antenatal classes. (After seeing the graphic film of a woman pushing and screaming in painful labour, I fainted, much to the amusement of my classmates.) The support of Emma and Richard and the uproarious laughter we created in class kept me sane during those very tense weeks after the accident.

Emma was determined to have a natural birth, but not me. To banish the labour pains, I wanted every drug available. I prayed that the baby would be fine and crossed my fingers for a caesarean delivery. As it transpired, my wishes were granted.

Thirty-six weeks into the pregnancy, the doctors noted that the baby was in the breech position. Due to the injuries I had sustained in the car accident and the baby's position, a caesarean was scheduled for two weeks' time, on my birthday, 29 July – and, spookily, my mother's.

Many of the nurses came to my health spa and toned their bodies on the gym equipment. One of the machines at the spa worked the pelvic muscles and had stirrups. How the two nurses laughed when they saw me being wheeled in on my back with my legs in stirrups after the epidural had been administered. 'It's just like working out at your health spa, Shelley!' said one of them. 'I hope it's as painless as that!' I retorted. The surgeons were curious about my spa,

and while they began the caesarean, the hospital staff and I
laughed and joked. My husband was horrified that I was
talking shop while on the operating table.

Tiny Rory (as we then called him) was born 10
minutes later at 38 weeks. He was thrust onto my chest,
looking like a baby alien. As I suspect many new mothers
are, I was horrified by his appearance. He was covered in
a mixture of yellow goo and blood, and had tufts of ginger
hair – an inheritance from his grandfather.

The nurses whisked baby Rory away to wash and
examine him. After being left alone for a while on a trolley
in the waiting room – the worst part – I was wheeled to
the maternity ward. It was only then that I was told that
Rory had been admitted to the intensive care unit for
babies. He had Respiratory Distress Syndrome, normally
a symptom of premature babies. This meant that his lungs
were undeveloped and he couldn't breathe unaided. Rory
had to be put into an incubator for artificial respiration.
I was told that Rory's Respitory Distress Syndrome was
most likely due to the fact that he hadn't grown much
in the womb since the car accident. He had all the
symptoms of a premature baby, despite being born at full
gestation.

I was the only mum in the ward with an empty crib
beside her bed – and I didn't feel like a mother. I felt
empty, as well as sore from the surgery, but I took delight
in the new babies of my fellow 'inmates'. It wasn't until I
was asked to express milk with an electric pump, so that
Rory could be fed with a drip, that I felt of any use. My
milk was frozen until Rory's tiny stomach developed
sufficiently to digest it, about ten days later.

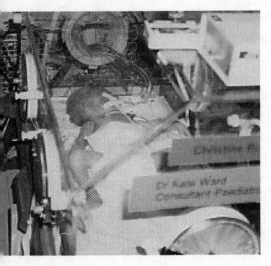

Baby Callum in the incubator – clinically confined!

On the day after the birth, I was wheeled into the babies' intensive care unit. It was so terribly hot inside the room where all the babies were lying in their perspex incubators. They were so small – some looked like skinned moles – and they were all wired up, with pipes and tubes connected to flashing and noisy machines. Rory was the size of my hand, pink and motionless. The tubes attached to him overwhelmed his tiny little body. I couldn't bear to stay for long – it was just too upsetting.

Shortly after the birth my husband announced that he didn't like the name Rory, in spite of the baby's red hair. He wanted to call him Callum, which was to be our choice if the baby was born blond. So Rory was now Callum. At the same time he announced that he wanted to sell our house because he didn't like his new, smaller office at home. (I had switched our home office to the smaller back room in order to create our new nursery for the baby.) I was surprised, confused and overwhelmed.

After spending ten days in hospital, I went home, leaving Rory in the intensive care unit. With the help of my husband's brother I redecorated the new baby room, despite suffering from the pain of the surgery, and changed it back into an office as a surprise for my husband on his return home that weekend.

One day I visited Callum in hospital, expecting to find him in the incubator, but instead one of the nurses was cradling him over her shoulder. Callum was so tiny and fragile that this was the first time since his birth that I had been able to hold him in my arms. I tried desperately to think of a nursery rhyme to sing to him – it's true what they say about losing your memory during pregnancy and just after birth! I ended up jiggling him around in my arms to the first song that came to mind, 'The Coconuts' by Kid Creole.

The first time I dressed Callum in his doll-sized romper suit, I didn't dare turn him over to fasten the poppers at the back. He was so delicate, and I felt ill-equipped to care for such a fragile, tiny baby. I was frightened I might hurt him. Of course the nurses soon had me turning him over and dressing him with confidence.

When we finally brought Callum home from the hospital in August 1992, it was with a mixture of excitement and trepidation. Callum was three weeks old and at this point he seemed to be a normal little baby. I was quite excited and nervous and couldn't wait to cuddle him in the comfort of our own home. I longed for us to be a proper family.

At home it became apparent just how small he really was. All the tiny clothes I had bought for him were way too big. He weighed a delicate 2 kilograms. Caring for

Callum left me utterly exhausted, and quite disorientated. It was as if I'd been out nightclubbing every night until 5 am. At lunchtime I was often still in my nightie, which was stiff as a board with dried breast milk.

After a week of breastfeeding and little sleep, I had broken every rule in the book. I had allowed Callum a dummy, or 'pacifier' as they're known in America, to help him settle, and he slept in our bed for his comfort as well as my own. Getting up to his cries in the night was physically and emotionally draining. My breasts would throb and leak every time he whimpered, so I never left him to cry.

I had also called the doctor out twice due to the baby's bowel problems. Because of his incomplete development

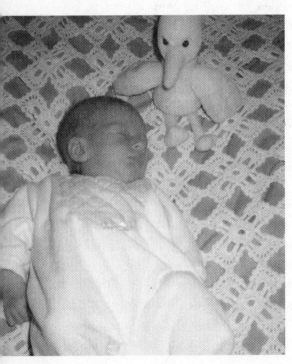

Callum on his first day at home, just 31 cm long, not much bigger than Stickle the Stork.

at birth, I was finding that Callum's stomach and digestive tract weren't functioning properly. During bouts of serious constipation, Callum's horrendous screams of pain were heartbreaking.

I could be metres away from him and still be able to differentiate his cry from a roomful of crying babies. I could also distinguish the meaning of his cries. I knew that if he cried a certain way it was a 'Mum, I'm hungry' cry, or an 'I'm tired and cranky' cry, and at other times there was the 'Help! I'm in serious pain' cry. The latter screams were the hardest to deal with. They were so piercing and lengthy that at times I could understand why parents sometimes lose the plot and shake their baby, or worse. It's so frustrating when your baby can't tell you what's wrong. My reaction was to burst into tears, which made Callum even more upset. The best advice I can offer for times of crisis is:

Always call someone for help, even a neighbour. You don't have to deal with the baby's screams on your own.

Sometimes I'd be beside myself at Callum's cries. I'd phone the doctor's emergency number so that he could administer an enema to relieve Callum's suffering. As time went by I learnt to balance his diet with liquid laxatives so Callum would have the chance to absorb nutrients essential for development. The stinky nappies were just the worst! One of the most dreaded aspects of being a new parent for me was changing poo-filled nappies. Life has a curious way of giving you what you don't want, in abundance … I was to have four and half years of nappy-changing, and still more years of accidents.

> Focus on what you want and not on what you fear.
> *Anthony Robbins*

With a little help

I was fortunate to have the support of a local midwife, who made daily visits during Callum's first week at home. In some ways this was stressful, because I felt that my home, the baby and I had to be clean, tidy and organised for the midwife's visit. I found it incredibly difficult to manage this, as I'd often had as little as an hour's sleep between breastfeeds. Sometimes I'd even vacuum the house at 2 am to catch up with chores before the midwife's visit the next morning!

On the other hand, it was great to have the midwife's reassurance that all was well with my delicate new baby. My husband was working away during the week on computer contracts in London or Leicestershire, but at weekends he tried to be an involved father. More often than not he looked exasperated, as I'm sure many new fathers do. My mother was very concerned about the baby and me, but as my friends from the antenatal class who had also just given birth were feeling equally exhausted, I put the tiredness and stress of coping down to being a new mother.

Nothing had prepared me for the demands of a new baby. Before Callum was born, I had no idea I would need so much support from family and midwives. Their confidence and serenity in the midst of chaos were very comforting. How on earth do mums manage to get ready in the morning, keep calm through screaming bouts, wash and feed the baby, look presentable for visitors, cook dinner, *and* stay awake? I had so many questions: Was I doing things right? Why was Callum sick? Why was he crying when he'd just been fed, washed and changed? The midwives who liked to take charge were a relief to me in my exhaustion. I gladly relinquished all responsibility at those times. How on earth would I cope when the visitors stopped dropping in?

The sudden loss of freedom entailed in becoming a mother was an enormous shock to me. I had never expected this little soul to be so time-consuming, and it was difficult having to do everything in my husband's absence. Like many mothers in the early days, I just wished for my newborn to say, 'Thanks, Mum.' A smile from this little boob-squeezing sucker would have been wonderful, but at first it's all take, take, take. And just when you think you can't give any more, the baby smiles or gurgles, and melts your heart. It's at that moment that many mothers and fathers feel that first connection of love.

At first I didn't bond with Callum in the way I'd expected. It took me a while to learn that most mothers don't feel deep pangs of love immediately. Many young mothers become depressed over their perceived failure to feel as they 'ought to'. I hope this book gives solace to any parent feeling guilty for not experiencing instant pangs of love for their baby. There is no set time for this bonding to occur, but I assure, you it *will* happen. For months after Callum's birth I was in a state of amazement that I had helped to create this beautiful little person. Even now I look at him and feel enormous awe and gratitude.

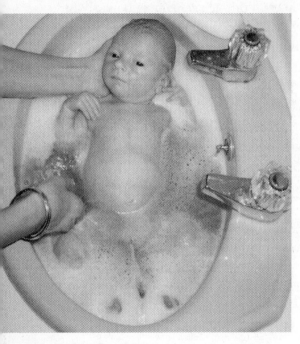

Callum having a bath in the sink. 'Oh boy, that feels so good.'

Early signs

When Callum was just a few weeks old, I could tell that he had a vision problem. He didn't seem to 'see' me, but he recognised my voice and his little face would light up when I spoke. All the baby books I had read stated that a baby begins to focus from the nipple to the mother's eyes from around six weeks onwards. I became increasingly concerned that Callum wasn't able to see. My husband dismissed my fears, saying that there was nothing wrong with Callum. My instincts told me otherwise. This strong intuition compelled me to take action and insist that Callum be referred to an eye specialist. It wasn't easy to convince the doctor, who tried to reassure me that many new mothers panic at the first sign of anything different. Eventually I cried and I refused to leave the surgery until he examined Callum and referred him to an opthalmologist (eye specialist).

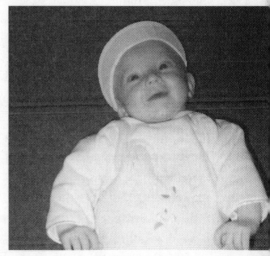

Callum not seeing but responding to Shelley's voice. 'I recognise that voice. Mama!'

Prior to the specialist's appointment, when Callum was ten weeks old, we took him to Switzerland to visit my friends Jenny and Martin, and their children, Keira and Schona. I had met Jenny and Martin in South Africa in my pre-marriage days. Jenny was Scottish and Martin was Swiss, and they had moved to his homeland to start their own family. Jenny was very spiritual and into holistic healing. She prepared some of her Bach's remedy to keep my energy levels high. She even suggested that they look after Callum for the weekend to give me a break and a chance to relax. However, Callum contracted a fever and was diagnosed with pneumonia.

The Swiss doctors were very concerned about his chances for survival. He was obviously vulnerable, so we flew straight back to England with him. I was utterly distressed, not knowing whether Callum would make it, so I organised a beautiful christening. In my anxious state I wanted it to be perfect. The small white church in Baildon, Yorkshire, where we held the christening, was similar to the church in the TV series 'Little House on the Prairie'. My Dutch friend, Sonya, flew over to be Callum's godmother. I lovingly made him a traditional christening gown and King Henry VIII beret from my mother and grandmothers' wedding gowns. On the day of the christening, 23 October 1992, Callum in his new family heirloom resembled a contented prince. The day went splendidly. Our family and friends rejoiced with us at the church and the reception that followed at Hollings Hall. Callum cooed contentedly as we cut the layer of brandy-soaked wedding cake that we had saved for the occasion.

Fortunately Callum recovered from the pneumonia. His first appointment with the opthamologist was in September 1992 at Bradford Hospital, when Callum was three months old. At the first appointment, the opthamologist confirmed that the baby wasn't seeing. After several visits to the eye specialist, finally a CT scan was recommended. A CT scanner consists of a large X-ray 'tube' housed inside a doughnut-shaped machine that rotates around the patient. The patient must lie absolutely still while the image is taken, so Callum had to be sedated.

Finally, after several long waits in the hospital, the opthamologist told me matter-of-factly, 'The good news is that Callum isn't unable to see due to eye defects, but because he has cerebral palsy.'

'Oh, that's wonderful news!' I exclaimed. Now I had hope. 'So what is cerebral palsy?'

'Mrs Sykes, cerebral palsy is brain damage.'

There is an order to the universe. In the midst of death, life continues; in the midst of untruth, truth continues; in the midst of injustice, justice continues; and in all darkness, there is light.

GANDHI

For the doctors who work with so many children with cerebral palsy, or more precisely, central spastic paresis, Callum was just another case. But I hadn't even heard of cerebral palsy – I could hardly even pronounce the words.

I can't recall racing out of the ward or driving home from the hospital, with Callum clutched close to my chest in his papoose. I was in deep shock … my baby wasn't just blind, he might end up a blind 'cabbage'.

My next memory is of sitting on my sister's doorstep, sobbing and hugging Callum tightly while mumbling incoherently. Nichola was really upset, having never seen me in such a distressed state. She knew it was serious, but she was also concerned for Callum's safety because

I was holding him so tightly, almost smothering him. I had geared myself up for the worst news about his eyesight, but there had been absolutely no suspicion in my mind that he was brain damaged.

I didn't know what to tell my husband, so I waited until he returned home that weekend. He listened but somehow couldn't accept that there was really anything wrong with his son.

Cerebral palsy

Cerebral palsy is caused by damage to the brain that occurs either before, during or soon after birth. 'Cerebral' means brain, and the term 'palsy' refers to the impaired control of body movements caused by brain damage. Often cerebral palsy is due to a lack of oxygen to the baby's brain during a difficult birth. Not all the causes of cerebral palsy are fully understood. It can be due to the mother contracting rubella (German measles) during pregnancy, a bleed in the baby's brain, a premature birth, a genetic disorder, or abnormal development of the brain that has no identifiable cause.

People with cerebral palsy are affected in different ways to varying degrees, depending on the areas of the brain that have been damaged. Someone with mild cerebral palsy might be clumsy or weak in their arm or leg movements, or their symptoms may be barely noticeable. Some sufferers have difficulties with fine motor skills such as writing, or with balance. People with severe cerebral palsy may have their entire body affected, making movement very difficult or virtually impossible. They may also suffer visual, perceptual, auditory or learning difficulties. Their concentration may be affected, and they may have trouble learning things instinctively.

Most families with a child with cerebral palsy aren't aware of it until the baby is several months old. It is only when the baby doesn't reach the usual developmental milestones, such as learning to support their head, roll over, sit, crawl, smile or walk, that the parents start asking questions. Most babies with cerebral palsy only show signs of the condition at around 12 to 18 months, when it's clear they're not developing at the same rate as other babies. At this time the baby's head might still be floppy, and they may not have begun to crawl or talk yet. It can come as quite a shock to the parents to learn that all is not well. But they are far from alone. Cerebral palsy is more common than many people realise:

Every 80 minutes in the Western world
a child is born with cerebral palsy.[1]
SPASTIC CENTRE OF NEW SOUTH WALES

According to the Murdoch Children's Research Institute at Melbourne's Royal Children's Hospital, 'cerebral palsy is the most common physical disability in children'.[2] Australian Bureau of Statistics figures quoted during Cerebral Palsy Week in 2001 in federal parliament stated that 'in Australia there are 20 000 people with cerebral palsy and of every 1000 babies born in Australia, between one and three children suffer from cerebral palsy.'[3] These statistics are shocking.

In addition, some of these babies are also born with other medical problems, including epilepsy, heart problems, skin conditions, breathing difficulties, and the list goes on. Hospital staff endeavour to support the families, but they encounter these conditions all the time and may have difficulty communicating sensitively, and in layman's terms. At first all a parent wants to know is exactly what's wrong, and what can be done about it.

In Callum's case, brain damage was caused by a lack of oxygen to the brain as a result of the car crash that I was involved in late in my pregnancy. My intuition about the cause of Callum's cerebral palsy was confirmed much later when further MRI scans proved that the damage had occurred between 32 and 34 weeks of foetal gestation.

At just three months of age, Callum was one of the youngest children diagnosed with cerebral palsy. The doctors told me that he was blind and had a bleak chance of ever getting out of a wheelchair. I didn't even know how to be a mother yet, never mind raise a child with special needs. How on earth would I cope? I couldn't bear to even think about it.

Miracles do happen. It's not what happens to you in life that counts, it's what you do about it that matters.

Life before Callum

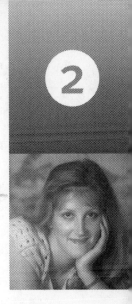

2

*An extraordinary life requires
mastering: the science of
achievement and the art of
fulfilment – the capacity to turn
dreams into reality, but also to enjoy
them thoroughly.*

Anthony Robbins

HAVE YOU EVER WONDERED why bad
things happen in your life, challenges that you never
wanted to face, but which you later realise were the best
things that could have happened to you? The hurdles,
once overcome, sometimes redirect your destiny,
putting you on a path that is more positive and more
constructive. It is during the trying times that many

people ask themselves: what is my purpose in life? I believe that the universal answer to this question is that we are here to love and serve others.

As a young woman starting out on life's journey, what I wanted from life was to be successful and appreciated, make a difference to people's lives, have fun, be healthy and happy, find and marry my soul mate, have beautiful babies, and enjoy financial security – not much to ask for!

My life has in actual fact been a series of adventures and disasters, interspersed with amazing luck, which has given me the strength to remain hopeful, to believe in and strive for my goals in spite of life's obstacles. The peaks and troughs seem to have been the universe's way of teaching me the lessons of life, making me the person I now am – someone who can touch, inspire and motivate others to follow their dreams and live a happy life, no matter what the challenges.

Until my son Callum was born, I had never really considered life in such simple terms as serving and loving, but I now realise that that is my true purpose. To explain how I came to take this path in raising my son Callum, I want to share with you something of my family background and the life I led before Callum was born.

My grandmother, Kathleen Hinchliffe, was born in Yorkshire, England, and orphaned at the age of four. She went to live with her aunt and uncle and their four boys, whom she helped to raise. At age 14 she met and fell in love with Thomas Haigh, a rather charming and good-looking manager at the local pin factory. They married when she was 23 and had four children, Ronald, Christine,

Stuart and Paulina. Unfortunately, Thomas found family life too dull and left Kathleen to cope on her own. Kathleen became the ultimate 'woman of substance', raising her four children as a single mother, establishing a fashion business and amassing wealth through property, including a street of houses.

Like my grandmother, my mother Paulina was a very creative woman with a penchant for clothes design, cordon bleu cooking, interior design and gardening, but she took the practical path of becoming a bank manager. My father, John, was a visual arts graduate, who also shared my mother's passion for design, but he left the arts world to move into the more lucrative business of telecommunications. Later, my parents set up two businesses, one in haulage and the other in diaries.

My birth in 1962 in Yorkshire was marked by two unusual things: I was born on my mother's birthday, as noted earlier, and I had two different coloured eyes, one blue and one brown (like the pop idol David Bowie). I was the first child in our family.

My younger sister, Nichola, arrived 18 months later, in March 1964. We were like chalk and cheese. Until the ages of 12 and 10 respectively, we were dressed in matching outfits, but our personalities were poles apart. I was the independent one, whereas Nichola was needy and demanded quite a lot of attention and support. I was quietly confident whereas Nichola was a shy child, who would hide under her arm.

I was fastidiously tidy, while Nichola lived in mess and disorder. Nichola shared my mother's prowess in the kitchen, whereas I would boil eggs until they exploded.

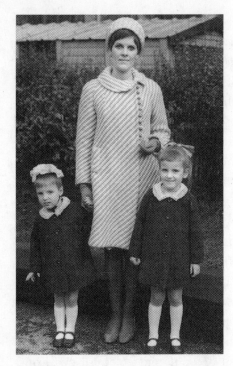

Nichola, Paulina and Shelley, 1966

We were brought up with an abundance of love, fun and affection, although the discipline was often strict.

Mum and Dad expressed their creativity by renovating old houses, selling them and then upgrading to begin the process again. It was a marvellous education for us. We moved house every few years and it was great fun.

Although I loved school, I wasn't as bright as Nichola, so I had to work really hard for my achievements. Nichola hated school but possessed natural talent. I was a 'Miss Goody-two-shoes' while Nichola was the rebellious one who pushed our parents to the limit. At grammar school no one could believe that we were siblings. My sister hated the fact that I was a boring 'swot'. She drank, smoked, swore and kissed boys, but she was always there to back me up if anyone tried to bully her older sister! Between us it was a real 'love you but can't live with you' scenario.

At the age of ten, I announced that I wanted to become a doctor, which came as quite a surprise to my parents. I had only just scraped into grammar school and was at the bottom of the class. My parents tried to prevent an inevitable disappointment by suggesting that I set my sights a bit lower and work towards becoming a physiotherapist. But Marie Curie, the physicist and chemist who discovered radium, was my role model. When my chemistry teacher, Mrs Cousins, said she thought I would make a great doctor, she inspired me to hold onto my dream. That's all it took – someone I admired who believed that I could do it. I learned to aim high and keep focused on my dreams. The belief that anything is possible has remained with me ever since.

Determined to improve my grades, I would walk to the school bus-stop with my nose in a book, totally engrossed. Nichola thought I was horribly un-cool. I'd work late into the night, reading, revising and doing homework, until Mum insisted I turn off my bedroom light. Eventually I bought myself a torch so that I could read under the sheets until the early hours.

All this hard work seemed to pay off. Three years later I won the school prize for the most improved student. It was expected that I'd get 'A' grades in my O-level examinations, the equivalent of the School Certificate in Australia. At the age of 14 when I sat the exams I got 'A's in six subjects, but I failed chemistry. It was an enormous shock to me that I had failed any subject, but particularly my favourite one. Mrs Cousins, my original chemistry teacher, continued to encourage me, and I managed to get an 'A' when I re-sat the O-level chemistry exam.

Back in the early 1980s, medicine was a popular university course. To qualify to study medicine, three A levels at 'A' grade were needed, and I only managed two Bs and a C. I was devastated. Some people would have considered these to be good results, but for me they represented failure.

I spent the summer of 1980 in France with my girlfriends, all of whom had scored three 'A's. In glamorous Monte Carlo, with my confident and go-getting personality, I was able to talk our way into places and situations you would only see in the movies. But inside I felt a failure, because I was focusing on what was wrong and not on all the great aspects of life.

I decided to re-sit the A-level exams. My parents couldn't bear to see me push myself so hard and go through all that stress a second time. They urged me to find a job rather than putting all that effort and energy into repeating the year at school. I refused to listen to them and left home, booking myself into a college that would allow me to re-sit the science A levels that I needed.

I had a Saturday job that just about covered my rent, and I lived off my savings. Thankfully I had inherited my grandmother's entrepreneurial skills. Over the years I had managed to save some money, because I had been working from the age of ten, doing paper rounds, babysitting, and even running my own brandysnap distribution business. I used to buy bags of brandysnap pieces from the local biscuit factory and sell the bags to my classmates for a small profit! I had also worked for Boots and British Home Stores, and had been a sales assistant for my grandmother's fashion boutique.

My fellow college students re-sitting the exams were mainly boys, so it was a completely different environment from the girls' school I had attended, where there were only four girls studying physics. Here the students' passion for the science subjects was much greater, which made the work seem easier. I was also able to take additional O-level subjects such as photography, art and design to release some of my pent-up creativity. The year just flew by.

The world beckons

After the exams, and while I waited for my results to arrive, I returned home to my parents and landed a fantastic, but poorly paid job with a travel operator. Promoting holidays and dealing with the customers was something I found easy, so I thrived in the work environment. After just a few weeks I was able to take my grandmother on a holiday to Malta and my sister to Majorca for her birthday.

I took every opportunity to fly at the weekends on the remaining undesignated flight seats to some European destination or other, once flying to Spain for the day for just £10, managing to do a spot of sunbathing, enjoying afternoon tapas, picking up some duty free for my parents and some beautiful clothes for myself, with a late-night dinner on the plane home. It was wonderfully exciting. These experiences sparked my lifelong passion for travel, for immersing myself in different cultures and ways of life.

In spite of working full-time, I felt that I should continue studying, so I enrolled myself in a part-time typing course and a journalism diploma course at the local university. Noting my professionalism, my employers gave me the opportunity to represent the company at several marketing events. At one of these events, a director of a chain of Spanish five-star hotels approached me to become the PR person for a new hotel in Tenerife. It sounded like a wonderful opportunity, with luxurious accommodation and an endless summer. At the same time, a job became available in the computer department at my firm. It was wonderful to have so much choice after just four months with the company.

Then my exam results arrived – they were exactly the same as my results from the previous year. It was bitterly disappointing, as my twelve O levels and four A levels were insufficient to study medicine. Instead of focusing on all the positive things I had achieved, I could only think of what I hadn't achieved. After all my hard work, I felt sure that my results would have improved. I couldn't help questioning why I had put myself through that extra year of studying. With hindsight I understand that I had wanted to do everything in my power to achieve the best possible results.

> Perfection isn't what life is about.
> It's the persistence of living that creates
> our greatest successes and joys.

My results were good enough to be offered a place at university to study pharmacy or chemistry, but I wasn't keen to do either. I really wanted to accept the PR position at the hotel in Tenerife, but my parents convinced me that I should use my qualifications to begin a career in IT. Hadn't their instincts been right in the past?

Reluctantly I began training as a computer operator, still working in the travel company. It wasn't as enjoyable as talking to the clients and travel agents, but the salary was better and I was still entitled to free holidays. However, I soon became restless, and felt the need to do further study. I applied to university to study IT full-time to become a computer programmer, and was accepted for the following year, 1981.

Being a bank manager, my mother placed great importance in financial security. My parents offered to give me a deposit for my first home for my eighteenth birthday in July 1980, or to treat me to a month's holiday in South Africa and a beautiful pair of diamond earrings. There was no competition.

> Happiness is found in doing,
> not merely in possessing.

The South African lifestyle, its people, the sunshine and the abundance of opportunities were enormously appealing to me. A woman I met during my trip told me that jobs in IT were far easier to come by in South Africa than England, because work experience was considered more valuable there than a degree. She recommended that I apply for work at the South African banks, as they offered ongoing training courses and would encourage me to do an Open University degree course. I loved the idea of doing my degree in South Africa, particularly as I could work and pay for my board while studying.

The day before I was due to leave South Africa, I typed up a résumé and made an appointment with the IT manager of a major bank. Mr Holt, an English expatriate, offered me a job and a contract so that I could apply for a visa to stay in the country. I cancelled my application for a university place in the United Kingdom, and six months later, at the age of 19, I migrated to South Africa. Comfortable in the knowledge that I was truly loved by my family, no matter where I decided to live, I had the confidence to set forth into the unknown. With my outgoing personality and natural networking skills, I felt confident that I would make new friends easily.

> Have the courage to leap into the unknown and take risks.

Life in South Africa

In October 1981 I arrived in Johannesburg. In South Africa's warm climate, and with my new-found independence, I soon flourished. The lifestyle was relaxed, and I found a beautiful white colonial mansion to rent with four others. It had a large kidney-shaped pool, a tennis court and a games room and bar that accommodated some wonderful parties.

The bank trained me to work on their IBM mainframes

as a network controller. It wasn't long before I realised just how tough it was for women in such a male-dominated world, but I persisted. I began my studies for an Open University degree through the Witswatersrand University and took a course in Cobol programming with Van Zyl and Pritchard, the top programming school at that time. I also studied Afrikaans at college. I would sit by the side of the pool and study, or take my books to read after windsurfing in the Vaal Dam. With servants to cook and iron for me, and access to a pool and tennis court, my new home was the epitomy of luxury.

The Zulu maids who looked after me were amazing women. Despite the apartheid regime, there seemed to be far less racial discord and resentment in Johannesburg than in Yorkshire, where skin colour seemed to bring out the latent racism in the locals. In Yorkshire in the 80s, black people were labelled as foreigners even if they were third-generation British-born residents. Most educated white South Africans I met at that time were of the opinion that people, black, coloured or white, deserved respect. However, I did notice that some Afrikaaner families had a rather condescending regard for the blacks. I remember one day in the city entering a lift where a black woman was on her knees washing the floor. She stopped when I got in and we exchanged greetings. At the next level, a boy of about ten years of age got into the lift and nonchalantly kicked the woman. I was shocked. The black woman just shrugged and seemed almost resigned to it. I insisted that he apologise to the woman, and it was his turn to be shocked.

Many of the racial troubles seemed to me to stem from the belief among the general white population that the black and coloured community was one body of people, when in fact it is made up of Zulus, Khosas, Northern Sutus and Swahilis, with each cultural group having its own distinct language and customs.

The blacks didn't seem to like the coloureds (part-black/part-white people), so they were treated differently again. It was sad to note that many wealthy blacks subjugated their own people in sweatshop work environments and bullied local black women into buying goods from their shops. One of my maids would buy goods from the 'white' supermarket and then have to take her purchases home tucked into her clothing, in fear of reprisal. I gave her clothes for her family, and she would wear them layer upon layer, on the way home, so that they would reach her family. Many black people were robbed by other blacks, especially the maids, since it was seen to be a privileged job with many perks, such as inclusive living quarters, free food, a good salary and gifts given to them by their employers.

The bank where I worked had very progressive employment policies, employing a majority of blacks and providing training opportunities for everyone. At that time, white women earned less than white men and the blacks less than the white women.

Years later it was wonderful to witness the abolition of apartheid in South Africa. However, it is very sad that so many of the uneducated blacks were promised the 'white man's way of life' for their votes, without understanding the economic consequences.

By the end of my first year in South Africa I realised just how much I felt at home there. I returned to England for a visit and was surprised at how little life had changed, whereas my life in South Africa had moved on in leaps and bounds. The buildings in England seemed small, dark and dirty, and the weather was cold and bleak, particularly in the Yorkshire Moors, near my family home. Despite my pleasure in seeing family and friends, it was such a relief to return to sunny South Africa.

In 1982, a year after arriving in South Africa, a wonderful opportunity came up to work for IBM if I was willing to do an MBA. The course opened up a whole new world of business to me. I found my niche in marketing and sales, specialising in selling system software to property developers and the manufacturing and distribution industries. I took up golf, because I thought it would be a useful addition to my business skills, and joined Toastmasters to improve my presentation and public speaking.

The thrill and variety of the business world and the financial rewards were very gratifying, but I really missed the travel industry. I was making inordinate amounts of money for someone my age, but I missed the excitement of travel and the opportunities provided by the travel industry. One day at a customer site, while speaking with one of the financial directors of a large company, I asked him what his dream was. He replied that he wanted to retire to the most beautiful place in South Africa, Knysna, where he and his family spent holidays. Only that week I'd seen a newspaper advertisement for a position as a director's assistant for one of South Africa's largest tour operators, Uniworld Tours. The role was to assist the CEO in all aspects of the business, as well as helping the operations and marketing directors to increase market share in

African resorts such as those in Knysna, the Drakensberg Mountains, the Okavanga Swamps, Botswana and Malawi. I certainly fancied travelling to those destinations.

I landed the job, but it was some months before I earned any free travel. Writing and producing the brochures for the tours to Asia and South America kept me busy. Before I started the job, I knew nothing about Asia or South America, but by the time the brochures were ready for print, I was longing to travel there.

Unfortunately this particular job wasn't the opportunity I had hoped for. I found myself quite isolated from the many office workers around me because, as the newcomer, I received many privileges to which my colleagues weren't entitled. As a consequence, my co-workers didn't trust me, fearing that I could be a possible snoop for the directors. In addition, my new Kiwi boyfriend, a computer engineer, had moved to Cape Town, and I was missing him terribly. In truth, I was miserable.

My girlfriends took me out to a nightclub one night to cheer me up, and somehow I managed to go on to win a national dance competition, with a prize that included a television drama course with the South African Broadcasting Corporation, as well as modelling and acting jobs in TV commercials, and money to donate to charity. My appetite for a career in the TV and film industries was whetted.

This win was a turning point. I decided to approach my company director about becoming the company's travel manager for Cape Town. The sales figures for Cape Town were the lowest of all the cities in South Africa, so I boldly told the company director that if I didn't increase sales in three months she could sack me! They offered me the job, but wanted me there in Cape Town that very weekend to host an airline presentation party.

I frantically packed and drove the 13 hours from Johannesburg to Cape Town, my little pink car full to the brim with clothes, books and photos, as well as the marketing material for the travel show. I had decided to surprise my boyfriend by showing up at his home. It was certainly a surprise for us both, as he had acquired another girlfriend.

What a nightmare! The only option was to plough my energy into my work, making friends with the staff of the 150 travel agents in Cape Town to increase the sales of holiday tours. My innovative plan worked. It was such fun to create free educational trips for the travel agents to Knysna, spending a whole weekend on the yachts, nature reserve and dining at the local restaurants. The fun and antics became legendary, and as a result we all bonded. The support the travel agents gave me was wonderfully rewarded with holiday booking sales. I was a tremendous success for the tour operator, and now in demand.

The yacht charter company later asked me to join them as their public relations manager in Knysna, a paradise where whales come to breed. My job involved taking tourists, who were mainly honeymooners, on the nature trails or out on a yacht, waterskiing or deep-sea fishing for marlin.

It was in 1986 that I contracted spinal and cerebral meningitis, as I briefly mentioned in Chapter 1.

I was flown by Red Cross ambulance plane from Knysna Hospital to Groote Schuur Hospital in Cape Town. I didn't respond to the usual treatments for meningitis – lumbar punctures and medication. Later the doctors informed me that it had been very touch-and-go for me in intensive care. Having contracted two forms of meningitis, and not responding to treatment, my chances of recovery had been very slim indeed. However, thanks to new drugs from the United States and with the care of top specialists, I was nursed back to full health. While in hospital, I realised how important it is to live life to the full and not worry about failure.

Life is too short, and while material things make life pleasant, it is the people we meet and our experiences that are the most precious possessions.

My brush with death gave me the impetus to leave Knysna to explore the rest of the world. My friend Patty, also a travel agent, had decided to live and work in Crete. I arranged to meet her there after a planned trip to Malawi.

Lake Malawi was mesmerising and I decided to stay on and work at the end of my two-week vacation. I began to teach snorkelling from a large catamaran on the lake in return for food and lodgings. The three months I spent at Lake Malawi were wonderfully liberating. I was able to swim with the hippos at sunset, and visit remote villages, where the women and children seemed to be fascinated by my long blonde hair. Of course, the fact that I had met a gorgeous 'Tarzan-like' man with whom to share the experience helped.

From Malawi I travelled on to Crete via Israel and Cyprus. At Aghios Nikolaos, a very pretty Cretan village resort, I secured a position as the PR and Entertainments Manager for a five-star hotel. For a couple of years I acted as the hotel's hostess to the United Nations, singing, dancing and entertaining the mainly European guests. It was brilliant – I worked for just nine months of the year and for the remaining three months I could travel. Another bonus was being able to invite my family and friends to stay at the resort. My dream of being a PR manager for a five-star hotel had been serendipitously fulfilled.

In 1988 I returned to England for my sister's wedding. Surprisingly, Mum and Dad were having marriage difficulties, and were just sticking it out for the wedding. This came as quite a shock to me – they had always seemed so in love, despite the usual marital grumbles. My parents had only ever seemed to fight about Nichola and me, or about finances. Mum was in emotional turmoil and the stress was making her ill. So I decided to move back to the United Kingdom to be near her, settling in Buckinghamshire, which was distant enough from my parents to maintain my independence.

In England I returned to start my own travel company and office machines business, but neither were as profitable as I had hoped due to the price-war going on, and so I revived my lucrative career in the IT industry, working for a successful software company. On the advice of my faithful bank manager, my mother, I bought a beautiful new townhouse.

Through work I met my future husband, Leigh, a Yorkshire man who worked in London as a programmer. I invited him to my house-warming party, where, to everyone's amazement, he just sat and watched the football!

Married life

Leigh and I had very different personalities, but he had completed a chemistry degree and worked in the travel industry before moving into IT, so we had a lot in common. I missed South Africa and, like me, Leigh was keen to live abroad in a warm climate. He was tall, blond and handsome and seemed to be an honourable fellow.

After just 13 weekends together, on a weekend trip to Gibraltar for his thirtieth birthday he told me that he had fallen in love with me, and then romantically proposed. I accepted without hesitation. At 26 years of age I wasn't sure what true love was, or whether it really existed outside of Hollywood, but I was sure that our future together would be a happy one.

Leigh and I shared some very romantic times. We had an amazing poolside wedding with family and friends at Las Brisas in Acapulco in May 1989, followed by a honeymoon in Cozumel. On our return to England, my mother hosted another wedding party for us at her farmhouse. It was a very exciting period in our lives. Our new home was being built in the village of Harden in Yorkshire. I was probably in love with the idea of being in love.

Leigh and I had discussed moving to South Africa, Australia or New Zealand, but he was dragging his feet and urged me to leave work as an IT consultant manager and start my own company so that I could spend more time at home.

Starting my own company seemed to be a good idea. In the previous months I had lost a lot of weight and become quite fit and toned, so that was my inspiration to establish a health spa. I had worked tremendously hard and passionately, producing some great results for the IT company. I had set up offices in Newcastle and been a trouble-shooter in Loughborough, living in hotels and travelling long distances, but producing impressive sales and establishing excellent business associations. The Yorkshire offices I had been asked to establish had been shelved several times and so I took the opportunity to discuss with my company directors my desire to begin my own health and wellbeing business. They agreed to let me take three months' unpaid leave to research the venture.

Honesty and integrity always seem to pay dividends.

I visited Switzerland and other spa centres to put together a business plan. My long-term goal was to franchise globally, beginning with salons in South Africa, Switzerland and Holland. My bank manger could visualise the big picture. It was a goer!

When everything was put in place, I opened the largest beauty salon in West Yorkshire, at that time. The whole enterprise took an enormous amount of my time and energy, but it was exhilarating. As the director of my own health spa, I developed a new passion for holistic healing and personal growth, and worked towards becoming a beauty specialist and counsellor. Within two years I was also given the opportunity to re-establish my TV career, becoming a news anchor, a professional speaker, appearing on radio and doing some acting work.

Some of the TV personalities I worked with became my health-spa clients. I was in my element, and my employees were very supportive while I went off to act, speak or be a stylist for celebrities and their homes. During this time my husband worked away mid-week on IT contracts. Opportunities flowed for me and I jumped at them. I managed to secure TV roles, including the role of dance partner to the husband of Catherine Zeta Jones's character in 'Darling Buds of May', a businesswoman in 'Emmerdale', village heart-throb in 'Heartbeat' with Nick Berry, and nerdy girlfriend to the lead in the BBC's 'Riff Raff'. Life was very rewarding and it seemed that I had it all.

It was during our third year of marriage, in 1991, that I surprised my husband by organising the holiday in South Africa, where we received the thrilling news that we were expecting our first child.

A mother's guilt

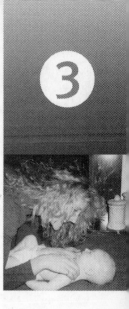

3

Every adversity, every failure and
every heartache carries with it the
seed of an equivalent or greater benefit.

Napoleon Hill

WHEN YOU LEARN that all is not well with your child and things haven't turned out the way you expected, feelings of confusion, disappointment, anger, self-pity, blame and guilt flood your mind. These are common and perfectly natural reactions.

When Callum was born and later diagnosed with cerebral palsy, my immediate reaction was to blame myself for having been in the car accident. Why was my baby hurt? Why not me? The more you pose negative questions, the more your brain produces negative answers. It can become a vicious circle if you let it.

> What lies before us, what lies behind us,
> is nothing compared to what lies within us.
> *RALPH WALDO EMERSON*

I didn't discuss my feelings with anyone at the time, or receive any counselling. Unfortunately, many new parents seem to have a real fear of appearing as if they can't cope. Yet none of us have been trained for the vitally important role of parenting.

No matter how much personal development I have done over the years, the negative feelings still pop up from time to time, but that's okay. I'm only human, after all. Being a naturally optimistic person, I gradually managed to pull myself out of the depths of self-pity and depression. I had to learn to accept that 'it just was' and ask better questions:

- Now that this has happened, what can I do about it?
- How can I transform a seemingly negative situation into something positive?
- How can I improve my child's condition and quality of life?
- What do I need to do first to make a difference?

The answers soon began to fall into place. By focusing on positive things, I realised that new possibilities arose. Immediately I felt better.

> There are no limitations to the mind
> except those we acknowledge.

The first lesson for me when Callum was diagnosed with cerebral palsy was to learn to rid myself of any guilt. The American psychologist Brian Tracy in *The Psychology of Success* calls it 'getting rid of the monkeys on your back'. This can apply to any area of your life: work, family, and relationships. Guilt is one of the most negative and immobilising emotions a person can experience. It helps absolutely no one and is more likely to lead to depression, bitterness and self-harm, both mental and physical.

With my feelings of guilt over Callum's cerebral palsy, I didn't need anyone else to make me feel unworthy. I was managing that all on my own. When self-criticism is added to the criticism that you inevitably receive from other people close to you, you rapidly lose the sparkle and magic that makes you who you are. Life becomes a huge burden to be endured.

My guilty feelings about Callum's cerebral palsy lasted for some time and then finally it occurred to me that I was wasting my energies and making myself miserable. I said to myself, 'STOP blaming yourself, Shelley.' It was clear to me that I had to be strong in order to give Callum the best chance of leading a 'normal' life. I realised the importance of looking after my own health, maintaining a balanced life and being true to myself, so that I could work magic in my son's life. I told myself that I had to be positive and bubbly, and shower Callum with unconditional love – all that anyone needs. Quite simply, I switched into pollyanna mode. 'Miracles happen, anything is possible,' I told myself. I declared that there was *no way* that my child wouldn't walk or be able to see. I promised myself, 'I'll do whatever it takes.'

> There is a powerful driving force inside
> every human being that, once unleashed,
> can make any vision, dream, or desire a reality.
> *ANTHONY ROBBINS*

The reactions of family and friends

When Callum was first diagnosed with cerebral palsy, family and friends didn't know what to say to me or what to do for me. They were as ignorant as I was about cerebral palsy, and most of them felt quite uncomfortable talking to me about it. From my experience, unless someone has a child with medical, emotional or behavioural difficulties, they can't comprehend your situation or know how to relate to you or comfort you. Everyone has an opinion, but often the opinion works in theory only.

Before we could find out the extent of Callum's condition, we had to wait to be called for a hospital appointment with the physiotherapist at the Child Development Centre in Airedale. Altogether we had three months of waiting, not knowing what action to take. Those weeks of not knowing how seriously Callum was affected by his cerebral palsy were the most arduous. I very much relied on my friends to keep me sane.

My three girlfriends, Emma, Sue and Alesandra, from antenatal classes, met with me once a week for drinks and cake. It was an excuse to dress up and compare our new babies, Bethany, James, Oliver and Callum, and their progress – the way they were smiling, eating, burping and so on. Our birthing experiences had brought us closer

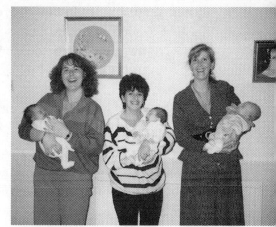

*Emma with Bethany,
Alesandra with Oliver,
and Shelley with Callum*

together and we clung to the friendship because of the shared feelings of inadequacy, uncertainty and curiosity that go with the territory of a new mum.

We laughed at the funny things we got up to in our new routines, and somehow supported each other when we were feeling ugly, exhausted and low. We had all assumed that after giving birth our bodies would spring back to their pre-pregnancy tautness, so we were all very disappointed to still look pregnant! Together we motivated each other to eat healthily. I encouraged the girls to work out at the health spa while their babies cooed in their baby seats nearby.

The support of my friends meant a lot to me. They accepted and liked both Callum and me for ourselves, not for what we had in life. They instinctively wanted to support me, and admired me for what I had to do on my own. All of them had supportive, loving husbands who enjoyed sharing the responsibilities of daily parenting, including getting up in the middle of the night to feed and change the baby. My friends' partners offered to help me if ever I needed anything, understanding that my partner worked away, which really touched my heart.

A father's denial

Sometimes a parent becomes resentful of their new baby because of the attention the baby gets. Many couples find a new child a threat to their relationship: they don't like having to share the affection, or they find a baby disruptive to the smooth order of daily existence. Having a child with special needs requires even more energy and time.

Callum's dad never accused me of being the cause of our child's injuries; in fact, he found it hard to accept that there was anything wrong with Callum at all, possibly because the responsibility was too much for him to bear. My husband didn't want to discuss the consequences that Callum's condition brought to our lives. As a woman, I thought it was essential to talk things over. My fears and concerns needed to be aired so that we could dispel them in a united effort. Instead, we locked our thoughts away, and any issues I raised were dismissed.

Negative thoughts flooded my mind. I felt ugly and at times was overwhelmed with boredom. I believed it must have been my fault that I felt this way. I really craved affection, love and support. I was so terribly lonely, even in my partner's company, and yet, being loyal and true to my husband, I didn't discuss my feelings with anyone.

It was also difficult with my husband only being home on the weekends. During the week I was alone with

Callum, and while I was happy with his company and our special routine, I still craved a cuddle and some understanding from my husband. But he had become very withdrawn, and he began to spend one weekend day at his parents' place.

By the weekend, when he returned home, I was desperate to get out of the house and have a normal adult conversation, but all he wanted to do was stay at home. He would offer to babysit while I went out. Sometimes I did attend functions on my own, which wasn't as much fun as it would have been with him, or I would give in and stay in too. The spark of admiration and passion between us had well and truly flickered out.

With my husband working away during the week, I spent a lot of time at home fretting over Callum. Also, my health spa business was suffering. I had two choices: I could sell it, or return to work to regain some normality and balance. I decided to return to work to re-focus my energies, for my sanity and my soul. And I was determined not to feel guilty about it.

I engaged a child minder, Brenda, who had been one of my clients and was renowned for her skills as a child carer. She was wonderful with Callum. She would put him to bed for his afternoon nap so that when I picked him up after work, I could do his physiotherapy exercises, and play and talk with him. It was a time when I was glad to be with my beautiful baby and he was full of energy. It was the perfect balance for us. Despite pressure from both families, who were concerned that I was putting work before child-raising, I knew that I was doing the right thing for my own spirit and, therefore, for Callum.

Secretly my friends admired me for standing my ground and following my heart rather than doing what others expected of me.

A marriage under strain

Women who suffer from postnatal depression, or men who feel they have suddenly become nothing more than providers, without the perk of sex, may generate guilt by failing to understand their own feelings. This, in turn, places unnecessary stress on themselves and their partner. Criticism is one way that they may chip away at their partner's self-esteem. Often the person criticising does so because they are unhappy with themselves. I was being besieged, but at that time I didn't understand why. Was I being too dramatic about Callum's health care needs, and was I a bad mother?

After all the criticisms, I was so concerned about my unworthiness as a wife and mother that I discussed my feelings, and the changes in my relationship with my husband, with my GP, who was horrified. He described how diligent and loving I had proved myself to be since becoming a mother. He confirmed that Callum's symptoms were genuine and would deeply affect us all, and that my diligence had saved Callum on several occasions. I was so relieved. It was lucky for me that I had asked for help and advice.

I decided from then on that my husband was responding in the only way he knew how, and wasn't able to communicate his feelings – I was not the problem.

I lived in hope that it was just a phase in our relationship that would improve with time. My husband worked hard and provided for us in the best way he could. I rationalised that he was just having a hard time bonding with Callum because he was away so often.

> No man is free who is not master of himself.
> *EPICTETUS*

Adjusting to motherhood

One of my earliest goals was to make Callum's life as interesting and enjoyable as possible. Because of his early blindness, Callum developed a keen sense of hearing and he just loved to be touched and comforted. So I carried him everywhere in a little soft papoose close to my heart, and played music whenever I could. The sound, movement and closeness to my body kept him quiet and content. He became less prone to crying. It is my belief that babies only cry when they are in need of something, so to leave them to cry – a habit from the Victorian era that seems rather out-moded and even cruel – is pointless.

Even at night I would bring him into my bed and comfort him after a feed. He would feel warm and content and snuggle up to sleep. Putting him back into a big, lonely cot would sometimes work, but if he wanted reassurance it would never do. As we all learn quickly enough, babies cry until they get what they need. My mother didn't think this was good parenting, but

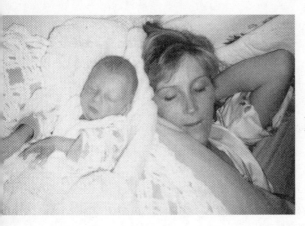

Life's tough – eating, sleeping, eating, sleeping ...

over the years I have spoken to many families who have happy, well-adjusted teenagers. The one thing they seem to have in common is never having left their children to cry, allowing them to snuggle into the parents' bed, even as they got older. Importantly, they even stopped what they were doing and picked the child up when they were obviously distressed, to comfort and reassure them. We have instinctively nurtured our children unconditionally.

We all get cross and frustrated – it's normal. However, it upsets me to see a parent ignoring their child trotting beside them with arms outstretched, distressed and screaming for attention. I want to shout, 'Please stop and give your child a hug and talk to them! Tell them why you're cross or tell them that their behaviour is unacceptable, but still hug them!'

A great parent loves unconditionally.

One step forward: physiotherapy

In November 1992, at three months of age, Callum was scheduled to start physiotherapy in order to better manage his symptoms. He had problems holding his head up, sitting up straight and grasping with his right hand.

At the Child Development Centre, Airedale Hospital, we were greeted by a smiling physiotherapist and a welcoming environment with plenty of toys for the children and caricatures on the walls. Ruth McAlister, the senior physiotherapist at the Child Development Centre, had been working with children with special needs for many years. Ruth explained to us that there are many degrees of cerebral palsy, with some children more seriously affected than others. She ascertained that Callum had all the signs of cerebral palsy – a floppy head, unresponsive and unprotective arm movements,

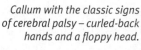

Callum with the classic signs of cerebral palsy – curled-back hands and a floppy head.

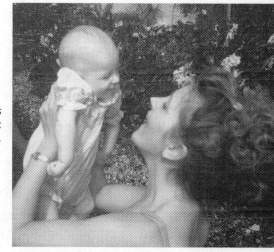

a lack of coordination and a lack of muscle tone in the legs and arms.

Ruth pointed out that Callum could have trouble walking, if indeed he ever learnt to walk, as well as many kinds of communication and motor-skills problems. However, she did recommend regular physiotherapy, based on a program designed by the Peto Institute in Romania, whose philosophy is that regular, repetitive movements to the limbs enable the brain to re-pattern and adopt normal functioning. We were told that the Institute's methods had made quite a difference to the lives of many children with cerebral palsy.

Lavish a child with praise at every achievement, no matter how small.

Ruth and her team were simply amazing. They were firm, yet gentle, and incredibly patient with each child. Leigh had come along on our first visit to the physio. It felt good to have him there and I was pleased that Ruth could demonstrate to him that Callum hadn't reached the usual baby milestones. She broke the ice with us by joking about Callum's pink vest (I had washed his white vest with my pink clothes by mistake). She also videotaped her session with Callum so that we could learn the moves she was demonstrating.

Some of the exercises Ruth performed made Callum cry, which was an unusual reaction for him, as he was generally a placid and happy baby, unless he was in pain. It made me feel sick inside. Callum found the exercises hard, but Ruth explained to me that if we didn't keep lengthening and stretching his tendons, his pain and discomfort would only increase as he grew. Callum's brain was sending signals to contract rather than relax his muscles.

Ruth impressed upon us that the more effort we put in now, the easier it would be for Callum in the long run. She did emphasise, however, that there was no guarantee that he'd be able to walk or move like other children. But without the workouts, he would certainly have no chance. My husband wasn't convinced that Callum was 'that bad'. As Callum was still just a baby, his development didn't seem too out of the ordinary, but I knew that Ruth was giving us an accurate prognosis.

During subsequent physio sessions, Ruth would assess Callum's degree of flexibility and run him through special exercises that I was to repeat at home. The exercises used equipment like plastic water-filled play bags that Callum would tap with his poorly developed arms to try and capture the brightly coloured shapes floating inside. Callum couldn't see the shapes, but he could feel them. Another exercise used revolving mirrors with bells on them, which would attract his attention. Ruth would direct Callum's hand to the mirrors. He would reach out and be surprised by the jingling noise they made as they rotated, which fascinated him. Callum was also placed on a sausage-shaped roller ball puff with his hands on the floor. He had to try to keep himself balanced, which was a real challenge for him. This exercise also helped to strengthen his weak back and neck muscles. Other simple exercises included aromatic massages, during which Callum enjoyed the sensations of smell and touch, plus stretching exercises. Whatever I was instructed to do with Callum, we did – and more.

We were loaned a special chair with sides to prevent Callum's head from flopping, and a low table that could be raised or lowered to the right height for Callum to be comfortable. We were also given a toy that could be suctioned to the table so that Callum could attempt to grasp it.

There was a long list of special toys for us to buy in order to stimulate his reach and touch and motivate Callum to produce responses that other children make instinctively. The beautiful highchair I had bought for Callum before he was born was suddenly out of commission, as was the baby walker. Apparently baby walkers reduce the movement of leg tendons, which is entirely the wrong muscle response to encourage walking. I sometimes wonder how manufacturers get away with selling equipment that physiotherapists tell us is in no way beneficial for babies.

All the beautiful soft shoes and leather moccasins I had purchased on my travels for Callum were no longer suitable. Instead, Ruth booked us in to see the hospital's foot and shoe specialist so that he could be measured for the cutest little red Spanish orthopaedic boots, and later AFOs (Ankle Foot Orthoses), which are plastic shoe splints.

Helping Callum learn to see

The other major battle that Callum and I faced was with his eyesight. Callum had acquired a severe squint from birth due to his cerebral palsy, and couldn't focus because of his eye muscles. It is quite common for children with cerebral palsy to experience problems with their eye muscles leading to a squint, but only rarely are they totally blind. I was informed that Callum could have an eye operation at 18 months to correct the squint, but that the surgery might not make any difference to his vision. I also learnt that a child's vision and brain patterns don't become fixed until the age of eight. In my mind there was still hope for Callum.

I decided to do whatever it would take to ensure that Callum had every chance of being able to see. Opthamologists recommended a strategy of eye-patching to strengthen his eye muscles. I would patch Callum's eyes daily with patches given to me at the hospital. Once a month Callum's eyes were checked for any vision improvement. We turned the eye-patching into a game. Some days Callum was a pirate, and on other days I would draw a picture on his dull, flesh-toned patch or I would place a sticker on it. Callum regarded it as normal to wear a patch, because he wore it every day.

I was determined that, in spite of his physical problems, Callum would benefit by travelling with us when we visited friends around the world. At the age of one we took him with us to Singapore, New Zealand and Australia. My husband had decided that it was the right time for us to move abroad. I was thrilled. He had a job interview in New Zealand with an IT company, so we booked our Christmas holiday to visit my South African–English friends in Melbourne before flying to Auckland.

It was just wonderful to be away together as a family, and it took my mind off Callum's impending eye surgery to fix his squint. The interviews went well and my husband was offered the job as an IT consultant in Auckland. He was to begin in April that year, 1994. We returned home and put the house and businesses up for sale. I agreed to stay in England until they were sold.

Eye surgery

Callum's squint was corrected when he was 18 months old in February 1994, just after we returned from our Australasian trip. Despite the doctors' warnings that it would make no difference to Callum's vision, I felt that if he was to have any chance of seeing, straightening his eyes to correct the squint would help.

For the sake of Callum's self-esteem, I also wanted the improvement that the surgery would bring to his appearance. Many young children have this operation at five years of age. By five, children know what's going to happen and the prospect of surgery frightens them. Also, their self-esteem may have already suffered through children teasing them at school and calling them 'squint eyes'. If I can offer any advice to parents it is to help your child look as close to 'normal' as possible. I really feel it assists them in so many ways, as it is one less problem with which they have to contend.

In spite of these motivating factors, I felt very anxious for Callum before he was to undergo surgery, experiencing nausea and fainting spells as the day of the

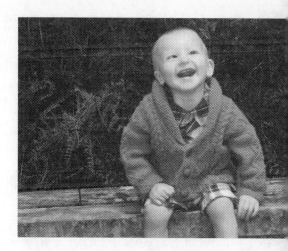

Cute but squinty. Callum aged 12 months, in Rotorua, New Zealand.

surgery drew nearer (my body's way of responding to severe stress).

I sensed that my husband was unable to handle the stress of our forthcoming move and of caring for Callum, so I kept my anxieties about Callum's operation to myself. Perhaps I should have tried to make more of an effort with our relationship, but he seemed to be so easily disgruntled. Instead I just tried to keep out of his way. I smiled and laughed a lot, as is my personality, but inside I felt drained. My mother sensed there was something wrong, as mothers uncannily do, and she was constantly nagging me to take better care of myself. It was tough.

When Callum went into hospital for eye surgery, I was given a camp bed next to his cot. I couldn't believe how many young children were waiting in their beds for the same operation, but were on their own. I became the 'Fairy Princess' of the ward, telling the children 'magical' stories. I also tried to impress upon them my confidence that they would all look handsome and beautiful after their operations. I brought bags of sweets for them that had 'magical powers' so that the injections would no longer hurt. The awe and wonder in the children's faces was worth every ounce of energy it took from me. Waiting for your child to undergo surgery is the most stressful time of all. I do recommend that any parent in this trying situation leaves the hospital to 'smell the roses' or do something positive for themselves, and if both parents can be there to support one another, the strain and understanding will be shared. I felt very isolated and alone. Staying in the hospital while your child is being operated on is simply too nerve-racking to endure. But children need you there for support and upbeat reassurance.

Callum returned to the ward sedated and with his eyes bandaged. By then I too was in need of a hospital bed just to recover from the adrenaline rush and intense feelings of anxiety! I collapsed into bed exhausted, but relieved that I had done the right thing for Callum. The operation had been a success and he no longer had a squint. Even though he still couldn't see, his appearance was much improved and I felt that he now had a better chance of seeing properly at some time in the future.

Somewhere, something incredible
is waiting to be known.
CARL SAGAN

Going solo

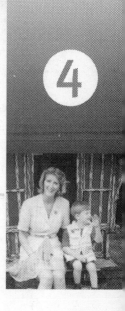

4

Talent develops itself in solitude;
character in the stream of life.

Johann Wolfgang von Goethe

BY EARLY 1994 our luck seemed to be changing. We had plans to live abroad once again, and not only had the eye surgery corrected Callum's squint but he was also making progress with his muscles. I was ecstatic after winning a trip to Hong Kong in a national hairdressing competition through work. I felt that Leigh and I really needed to enjoy this holiday together as a couple, especially after the anxiety of the eye surgery. A week on our own – how wonderful! Callum's nanny, Brenda, offered to look after him for that week. I couldn't wait to tell my husband that evening.

But I was stunned when Leigh told me he wasn't interested in going. He explained that it was because of work. Then, after my many suggestions to remove that obstacle, he finally revealed the real reason: he wanted a divorce.

> All truth goes through three steps:
> First it is ridiculed. Second, it is violently opposed.
> Finally, it is accepted as self-evident.
> *ARTHUR SCHOPENHAUER*

I felt as if my world had just collapsed into a black hole and I was in free fall. I ended up taking the trip with my mother, who was a great boost to my spirits at this upsetting time. She reminded me of who I really was.

My husband had looked elsewhere for solace. The combination of working away from home, the strain of a special-needs baby, our personality differences and my lack of perception in our relationship had culminated in our separation.

Tough as it was, I was relieved that Leigh had had the guts to tell me, to leave and not keep living a lie. I deserved to be loved unconditionally and be part of an uplifting partnership, and if that wasn't possible with him, I could at least be free to share my life with someone who'd appreciate me. I had no regrets about our marriage, because I had the most beautiful child and had gained a wealth of knowledge about relationships.

That's not to say that I wasn't very emotional about

our marriage breakdown. As you can imagine, losing my partner to someone else really knocked my confidence. I took it personally.

My lesson from these experiences is to keep the romance in your partnership alive and keep loving your partner, especially after childbirth.

Adjusting to parenthood

Coping with exhaustion and stress is one of the major challenges we face in our lives today, especially when combining general life issues with having a baby. For parents of a baby with special needs there is the added strain of dealing with the baby's particular health problems.

We can all make excuses. Exhaustion makes you grouchy and irritable. How can you be sexy and fun to be with if you don't do things that make you feel sexy and fun? Take time out and have naps, do things that you like, and create a happy, loving home. And heed these wise words from the Dalai Lama:

The best relationship is one in which your love for each other exceeds your need for each other.

Tiredness, stress, exhaustion, disappointments, the unknown – all of these contribute to new parents feeling unattractive and unromantic. For most women, particularly if they had a bad time giving birth, the last thing they feel like is being romantic with their partner. They may even express their frustration in a hurtful manner. But remember, poor dad can often feel just as tired as mum. He too is woken up in the middle of the night by the crying baby, yet he isn't able to do as much for the baby as the mother, especially if she is breastfeeding. It is a very emotional, intense time, a time when the mother needs reassurance that she is doing a great job as a mum and is still the most beautiful woman, and a time when the father needs to hear that he is still very important and very much loved.

It's worth going that extra mile to show the ones we care about how much they are loved. The romance shouldn't stop when you become a parent.

I missed this most important lesson in relationships, despite my mother's advice. I think we expect our partners to know instinctively that we love them and appreciate them. Unfortunately, I was a late learner. I can assure you, we all need to be told that we are loved, and shown love with consistent gestures.

A great partner shares the responsibilities of being a parent, and still finds time for their partner.

A single-parent family *can* manage the rigours of raising a child, but keeping the family happy and united will save you a lot of heartache. It is so very important to remember that we are on this earth for just a very short time and we owe it to ourselves firstly, and then to our partners, to be the happiest we can be. If you feel happy and fulfilled, your children will also be happy. And if you're happy, your partner is more likely to be content too. And if your partner is unhappy, then he or she is the only one who can change that.

To keep your relationship strong after the birth of your child, give yourselves the chance to live life to the full:

- Organise a weekend away together, or a night out with friends, not as parents but as a couple. By doing this you are more likely to feel like you are living and loving rather than just existing from day to day.
- Remember to keep the sparkle of romance in your life so that you can love generously. Make a habit of regular, simple, thoughtful acts towards your partner.
- Your child will benefit by gaining the perspective that family life is full of love. They'll appreciate you and the things you do for them all the more if they feel secure and loved at home. No one else can ever teach your child how to love in quite the same manner as you can.

In a partnership you need to feel as though you are living as an individual as well as a couple.

If, in spite of all your attempts to keep the romance alive, your relationship breaks down, try to come to terms with it (seek counselling to assist with this process, if necessary) and be civil and honourable to your ex-partner for the sake of your children. Too many adults use their children to hurt one another, which torments the children, lowering their self-esteem and confusing their understanding of love and loyalty.

Legacy of a marriage breakdown

For me, the marriage breakdown left me in terrible financial straits: I had been left with debts and empty savings accounts. I was emotionally and financially devastated. Callum and I had been left so poverty stricken that I couldn't even afford to heat the house. We would climb into my bed wearing layers of clothes and a coat. We'd snuggle up and I'd spend hours reading Callum happy-ending stories.

It took the Income Support Department – the British state welfare – six months to come to our rescue. Fortunately, they allowed me to keep my business rather than go bankrupt because I assured them that I could rebuild a cash flow and ultimately not be dependent on state benefits.

It's not what happens to you in life,
it's what you do about it that counts.
W.M. MITCHELL

I could no longer afford to retain the gardener, the ironing lady or Brenda, Callum's nanny. I opened a crèche at work so that Callum could be with me while I continued to manage my business. To the outside world everything seemed okay: I was still living in the house, I had the business running on a week-to-week basis, and I paid the staff salaries from the cash coming in. But I had lost weight because I couldn't afford to eat properly. The mounting bills and debts left me with very little.

I felt an overwhelming guilt that I had failed Callum on two major counts. Not only did he have to contend with his disabilities, but he was now the child of a broken home. I was at my lowest ebb. Just when you think things can't get any worse, something else always seems to happen to prove you wrong!

> Our greatest glory is not in never falling,
> but in rising every time we fall.
> *RALPH WALDO EMERSON*

Money is a wonderful asset – just another form of energy, really. However, many people place money above love, honour and integrity. We have all heard stories of women taking their husbands 'to the cleaners' and using their children as levers for money. Equally, we have all heard about men who have left their partners with the sole responsibility of raising the children. I think highly of any man or woman who does the honourable thing of supporting their children emotionally and financially after the disintegration of a relationship.

For twelve weeks Callum and I had to attend the child protection courts to sort out the custody of Callum, which now, strangely, seemed to be linked to the ongoing court case following the car accident and Callum's cerebral palsy payout (still in progress today). It was frightening to think that I might lose custody of Callum to my ex-husband. It was unimaginable – losing my baby ... Fortunately for me, my very best school friends, Jacquie and Jean, supported Callum and I in their own special ways, as did Brenda our former nanny, the doctors and my solicitor. It is true that you find out who your real friends are in times of need. I was in a constant state of shock and despair; I had lost my will to fight. I was ready to run away with Callum.

On the day of the court hearing I was in a very emotional state. I couldn't bear the thought of losing Callum because of a judge's decision, so I grabbed a suitcase and fled with Callum under my arm to the local airport, Leeds/Bradford. We caught the first flight out ... it was to Corfu. I had always fancied the spontaneity of arriving at an airport and just deciding my destination on the spot, but not under these circumstances.

Running away with Callum like that was an irrational act, but I felt desperate. After phoning Jacquie in England to find out the verdict, I spent the first day in Corfu crying with relief that the courts had ruled in my favour. I had won custody of Callum. It was fortunate that the judge wasn't aware that I had run away: it certainly would have been frowned upon, and I wouldn't recommend anyone taking that course of action.

A child's pain

I've never regretted marrying, nor have I felt bitter about the circumstances of our marriage break-up, because I had my gorgeous baby son. Acrimonious divorces are common, but the saddest thing is that it's always the children who suffer the most. The stress of the divorce certainly made me sick, and Callum too has been affected by the events. As a result he has had to have many sessions with psychologists over the years.

After the separation and divorce, Callum lived with me and spent every alternate weekend and alternate Christmases at his father's house. Callum would go to his father's new family home on the Friday nights and then to his grandparents on Saturdays when his dad went to the football, returning home to me on Sunday mornings.

Callum's behaviour after weekend visits to his father became challenging. When he got home, he would weep or become angry and aggressive with me. I didn't understand why. He wouldn't let me hug him or kiss him for most of the morning, nor would he tell me why or what had happened. He would injure himself by banging his head against the wall in frustration, or he would burst into tears. Money seemed to play a large part in his anxieties. He would regularly ask me when he returned from his weekend visits who paid for things, something most children are not aware of until they are eight or nine years of age – Callum was just two. Callum's preschool teachers would often phone me on the Monday to say Callum was upset.

It wasn't all bad. Callum loved his paternal grand-parents, baking with his grandma and doing woodwork with his grandpa. He also loved telling everyone he had a new stepbrother and step-sister.

However, one day it dawned on me that if anything happened to me, there would be no one to take Callum through his daily physiotherapy exercises. Who had the passion and determination to help him to reach his potential? I had to look after myself to ensure that I was around for Callum. There was no one else from either family who could love him as I do – no matter what.

From that moment on I was determined to be a mum like no other and to raise Callum by following my instincts and learning as much as I could.

It's in your moments of decision that your destiny is shaped.
ANTHONY ROBBINS

Callum needed support, and so did I. His tantrums after weekends with his dad were completely out of character and I had no idea how to deal with them. Beside myself with worry, I requested support from a psychiatrist through the Child Development Centre. Callum under-went a series of psychological tests, including games to check his motor skills, self-esteem, comprehension, perception, spatial-visual skills, communication, as well as psychological analyses with regard to his perception of his disability and his understanding of his parents' separation.

One of the first questions the psychiatrist put to me was whether I had discussed with Callum the reasons for his father leaving. Had I explained to him that he, Callum, wasn't responsible? I was shocked. My answer was, 'No, my baby is too young for that. He's only 20 months old.' But the psychiatrist explained that from a very young age children can tell if there's something wrong at home. They will often blame themselves if the parents don't explain what's happening in a language they understand. This was my first important lesson in child psychology.

Children need to be kept informed of situations that affect their lives, no matter how young they are.

Needless to say, that afternoon I sat with Callum and explained to him what was happening between his father and me. Callum's reaction was quite amazing to me. He seemed to accept my explanation and, gradually, with the assistance of the psychologists at Airedale Hospital, Callum's behaviour after the weekend visits to his father improved a little. The psychologists were brilliant, and I credit them for much of the knowledge I have gained. They recommended that it was better for Callum to continue his fortnightly visits to his father's family, despite the adverse reaction he displayed after these visits. The psychologists suggested that Callum was protecting me and didn't want to upset me by revealing his feelings (although his sadness was quite apparent to me).

The psychologists taught me how to handle the distress and how to reaffirm my love and affection. They were so marvellous, but it was hard to watch Callum's change in spirit after his weekends away. The disruption to his routine and the change in family environment appeared to take their toll on him, and his anger and frustration were reflected in his behaviour. I came up with a few strategies to help Callum overcome his low spirits after these visits. I would arrange for an exciting trip out when he returned home, or would invite his friends to come over. It helped to relieve the pent-up frustration.

I devoured every self-help book I could get my hands on and worked to rebuild my own self-esteem after the marriage collapse. There was only one way for me to go, and that was up! I wanted to stop feeling like a victim of circumstance and regain control of my life.

If I was to help Callum, I had to build myself up to be the happy, bubbly, positive person I had been before all of these troubles had reared up. As they say in those in-flight safety demonstrations before a plane takes off, 'secure your oxygen mask before fitting a mask to your child'.

I was determined that Callum would have every opportunity that he would have had if my marriage hadn't fallen apart. I wrote down my objectives and dreams for Callum:

- be happy and sociable
- learn to see
- learn to walk
- travel the world

I then wrote down my own goals:

- be healthy and happy – a woman like no other
- meet a gorgeous new man
- achieve financial freedom
- travel the world
- revive my TV career

I didn't know how we would achieve these goals, but I was determined that we would succeed.

> Nothing splendid has ever been achieved
> except by those who believed that something
> inside of them was superior to circumstance.
> *BRUCE BARTON*

The Hand of a Friend

The hand of a friend is a hand indeed
Holding the key to life's treasure
Like the sun that is golden,
Like a harvest of seed,
Clasp it well, grasp it tight,
With its measure of warmth and love,
Bringing you joy to the heart
Friendship, like a long winding road,
Wander down quietly, then you can start
Recalling the moments what 'ere the mood.

Happy days, sunny days, laughter and tears,
This hand of a friend like pure gold,
Never to tarnish, nor lustre fade
Gives strength as the memories unfold,
When everyday life which relentless evolves,
Treasure the friend who lightens the load
Take the hand, grasp it well, the problems resolved.

In the quiet of evening, when birds are hushed
The fragrance of flowers fills the air,
Think of friends, who may be far away,
Though the miles of thought bring them near,
Sleep peaceful as dawns another day
Bringing knowledge that when you have need
There's a hand of a friend, faithful and dear,
A smile on your face will show the world
You hold the hand of a friend indeed.

SYLVIA G. POORE

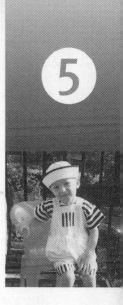

From the outside looking in

*The vision that you glorify in your
mind, the ideal that you enthrone
in your heart: this you will build
your life by, this you will become.*

James Allen

SUPPORTIVE FRIENDS AND FAMILY are
a wonderful asset. They can relieve the pressure from you
and your partner by giving you time for yourselves. They
can help with babysitting, and be there to support you
emotionally when you are upset, confused and feeling down.

But family and friends can just as easily be a negative
influence in your life. They may have preconceived ideas
as to how you should raise your child. Perhaps they frown

upon you taking time out to relax and have fun. Maybe they don't agree with your decisions for your child, or they worry about what other people may think.

I find it helpful to keep the following thoughts in mind:

- If you're lucky enough to have a few family members and friends who make you feel good and have a positive influence, keep them around.
- Distance yourself from anyone who bullies you or makes you feel depressed, no matter how much you may love each other.
- Only you know what's right for you, your child and your family. Advice is all well and good, but we have our own lessons to learn in life.
- Sometimes the journey of risk, adventure and learning makes life worth living. Criticism can bring you down and cause you to lose confidence.
- Don't waste time trying to please everybody. Keep yourself happy and healthy and trust your instincts.

My family is very loving and expressive, which is wonderful until you disagree with their way of doing things! I'm sure many people can relate to the Greek family portrayed in *My Big Fat Greek Wedding*. The father of the family assumes that his daughter will marry a man of Greek background, have babies, and forego forging a career. This film is a memorable depiction of the restrictions parents can unwittingly place on their children.

My mum, lovingly called Klucky by her grandchildren after a character in Walt Disney's *Robin Hood*, was always hugging and kissing my sister and I when we were little.

She now extends this same love to her grandchildren. She bakes and brings out the paints, jigsaws and videos galore to entertain them. Klucky was the catalyst for giving Callum the inspiration to want to run when she showed him the *Forrest Gump* video when he was four years old.

My sister's family has always included Callum and have often invited him to stay over and attend parties. My niece Amber doted on Callum from the very beginning, and even now the cousins, Amber, Sebastian and Callum, are very close. Children always seem to know how to love unconditionally, and Callum's cousins are no exception. They have always enjoyed helping me with Callum, and being unconventional (I'm Princess Shelley, not Auntie Shelley), it was fun for me to dress them up in tuxedos, suits and party dresses and take them out with me whenever we got the chance. Children love adventure and to feel special and important.

Sometimes family members can't cope with particular situations. My mother, for example, found it very hard to see Callum having physiotherapy. She is squeamish. She would shout at me not to hurt him, which would really upset me. The last thing I wanted to do was hurt my baby! Mum was still working full-time, and understandably she found child-caring at the weekends hard, especially with Callum because he wasn't toilet trained and was prone to bed-wetting, falling, and other accidents, which were part and parcel of any stay. A few hours were much easier for her to cope with, and I understood that.

Mum and my sister have very definite, conventional views of how to raise a child. Also, they are both cordon bleu cooks and are passionate about food and cooking. I was hopeless in the kitchen, so salads and microwave dinners were my forte. Their criticisms and jibes would make me feel bad about myself, at a time when unconditional encouragement and support were what I needed most from them. I knew I was doing the right thing for my child, but their criticisms made the job much harder.

By distancing myself, I was able to keep my spirits high and get on with caring for Callum without being made to feel as though I was in the wrong. I realise that no one was at fault here. My family loved both Callum and I, but I knew I was doing the right thing with Callum's physiotherapy to give him the best chance of walking.

> By knowing when to keep your distance, you can avoid conflict and remain friends with the ones you love.

Social consequences

When Callum was just a baby, nobody ever really discussed his symptoms, because they weren't noticeable. Socially, things went well for us. Because Callum was so content and docile, everyone would coo and marvel at his good behaviour. Nobody noticed that he couldn't see, crawl or walk.

As Callum got older his physical problems became more noticeable. Many people don't feel comfortable around someone who looks different. Callum would either be ignored completely, or they would talk as if he wasn't there. Fear becomes a big obstacle to social interaction – the fear of doing or saying the wrong thing. But really, we should all just be ourselves.

Also, friends and family often worried about something going wrong while Callum was in their care. Parents expect their child to trip or fall a lot, but outsiders care so much that the last thing they want is to have an accident with your child.

I understand that accidents happen, particularly to Callum, due to his poor mobility and balance. The reluctance of friends and family to have Callum stay over at their place was very hard to accept, but I tried not to take it personally. They simply didn't want the responsibility.

> Recruit assistance only from friends, family or agencies who are genuinely willing to help out. Why? Because your child will pick up the vibes very quickly if they're not truly wanted.

Bed-wetting, toilet accidents, bumps and falls are routine to any child, especially those with special needs, so I had to learn to deal with these things without anger or frustration. When at times it all became too much, I didn't become reclusive and try to manage it all on my own. I recognised that I needed to recharge my batteries, and so I turned to the many agencies offering support, such as 'Give a Mum a Break' in the United Kingdom, or club membership weekends through the Spastic Society in Australia. Local councils also provided babysitting, help, advice and occasional childcare. Even if it was just for one or two nights, it was important to take this time out. I realised that for my sanity I needed outside help. 'Give a Mum a Break' linked me with the most loving, happy family, the Owens. They had been trained in caring for special-needs children, and their house had been fitted with special protective gates, bed bars and so on. They wanted to make a positive difference, and what a godsend they were to us.

Sharon and Anthony Owen have two children, Lucy and Jamie, who have red hair. They just took to Callum, and with his red hair Callum looked just like one of the family! He would stay over at their house if I had to work or if the weekend with his father had been changed or I was really stuck for help. For Callum it was great because he was treated like a best friend. He got to experience a normal, happy family environment. Anthony was a great father role model. Sharon and Anthony shared my philosophy for raising children – leading by example. They brought contrast and balance into Callum's life. Callum was able to see the differences between family life with the Owens, family life at his father's and life on his own with me, and to experience the benefits of life in each family.

The gift of loyal friends

At some stage in our lives we all feel like victims, and sometimes we allow ourselves to be used and abused by people who expect things in return for their friendship. Often these very same people don't stay around long when the friendship is needed most.

How to pick and attract friendships where there are no expectations, just the enjoyment of one another's company, is something worth learning.

I have always been blessed by attracting some of the most wonderful people into my life, as has Callum. Thanks to them I've been able to get through a very hectic schedule of childcare, working, hospital visits, charitable work and, of course, partying and holidays. Many doctors and physiotherapists have become friends around the world. My clients and staff have been just fantastic – they have kept me on track, helping me get where I needed to be each day, because I was so involved and passionate about my work helping others to achieve their goals. I had such a full diary. If Callum was sick, my staff worked overtime to help me, and the clients were wonderful about it. It made my working life so much easier … the hours, days and weeks just raced by.

The love bestowed on Callum by his carers – his nanny, Brenda, and her boys Sam and Ross, Jeanie and Peebo, the Owens family, Callum's support teacher Rachel and her family, Tony and Jay, just to name a few – gave me the freedom to create a new life for Callum and myself. We were like 'the A team'. My friends were so loving and supportive, sometimes by simply offering a listening ear or generously sharing parties or holidays with us. Most importantly, we shared a great deal of laughter.

By surrounding myself with loving, generous friends and family I have been able to maintain the momentum of self-love and unconditional love.

We choose our friends and they are attracted
to us for our energy and who we are.

I find that the right people seem to come into my life at the right time. There are those people you meet who you feel as if you've known for a lifetime, who are like soul brothers and sisters. True friends are the people who accept us just as we are. Where the respect between friends is mutual, the energy just keeps revolving and boosting us to higher levels.

It is the people in our lives
that make our lives literally worth living,
and not the things in life.

Making Callum's exercise program enjoyable

Over the months and years of weekly physiotherapy visits to Ruth McAlister and her team at the Child Development Centre at Airedale Hospital, I received so much support, for which I can hardly thank them enough. After the initial visit with my husband, it was tough taking Callum to physio on my own. Even finding parking in the hospital car park was stressful for me at that time. Ruth told me it wasn't surprising to see me on my own, as she explained that 90 per cent of marriages where there is a child with special needs end in divorce. It was almost a relief to hear that mine wasn't the only marriage that had cracked and crumbled under the strain. People everywhere were obviously suffering.

Ruth was very supportive of my unusual interpretation of her exercises for Callum. When she asked me to open his legs and push down on his inner thighs 20 times for three sessions, to me it sounded dull, painful and boring. Callum's grimaces and cries were also painful to me, so I invented fun ways of completing the exercises. For example, I would open his tight thighs and put them around my hips, then dance for several minutes. Callum loved my singing and dancing and being swung around. Although it hurt, he didn't know whether to laugh or cry, but most times he would laugh. During the sessions of opening and pushing on his thighs, I would be sure to tease him by blowing a big raspberry on his tummy. He would laugh at the sensation and the farty noise I made!

The best way to approach anything unpleasant or difficult is to make it fun.

One aspect of the physiotherapy was to strengthen his back and bend his knees to teach him the sensation of crawling. I spent hours bending his knees and holding them in place. I even got cramps in my hands, just so that Callum could feel what it was like to crawl. The independence my little Callum gained by being able to feel what it was like to crawl gave him the determination to want to do more. A normal child learning to walk won't quit until he or she can walk, and nor was I willing to quit until Callum could crawl.

Ruth gave me the courage to try fun, new games and to feel confident about the way I was raising Callum. She gave me a great deal of positive feedback, and there were many signs that Callum was making incredible improvements compared with other children with cerebral palsy. I was inspired to keep motivated and persist, gaining confidence in myself and in my intuition. I believe that a parent does instinctively know what is right for their child. Ruth supported me every step of the way and never once dampened my enthusiasm.

> Imagination is more important than knowledge.
> *EINSTEIN*

The author of *Think and Grow Rich*, Napoleon Hill, has a son who was born without ears. Napoleon and his wife decided that they would treat their son as if he could hear and helped him to live a full life, despite the obvious setbacks. Napoleon had a gut feeling that somehow his son would discover a way to hear. The 'cure' or miracle came through vibration. Napoleon's son loved to hear music through vibrations, so he would lay his head on the sideboard holding the stereo in order to hear the music. As a result, new hearing aids were developed using vibrational technology. Napoleon's son now tests hearing aids. He also gives motivational talks about his life and career.

Every day I'd spend hours with Callum doing various tasks to help him overcome his symptoms. Inspired by my experiences with massage and other alternative therapies, I tried speaking directly onto his arm so that he could feel the vibrations from my lips. I believe that the sensation of my lips speaking on his skin over time stimulated a neurological re-patterning that helped with his speech development. I am certain that all these tasks activated different areas of Callum's brain to speed up the development of his speaking skills. His first official word was 'picture', and then, of course, 'Daddy' and 'Mama', but by nine months old he was speaking in comprehensible sentences and surprising people. It is said that most people who are disadvantaged in one aspect of their life evolve sharper senses and strengths in other areas. For example, blind people develop an acute sense of hearing. This was true for Callum.

I would also massage Callum's little body for at least an hour daily and support him on my hip while doing chores or dancing around the house. He loved music and being touched, so I made this part of his routine. Many of the exercises, and the routine of stimulation and play that we undertook, were simply improvised by me. Having an active and vivid imagination, I was willing to try my own methods in conjunction with the expert advice given to me by the physios and other therapists treating Callum. I certainly encourage parents to invent their own games and exercises for their children. After all, we are all blessed with limitless imaginations. This play time is so very important for all children.

Imagination rules the world.
DISRAELI

Many of the parents at the group physiotherapy sessions became disillusioned when told that their efforts there might not make a great deal of difference to their child's development. However, what I realised was that one hospital physio session per week really isn't enough for a growing child with spasticity. Every day counts. Like a gym workout, you don't achieve a toned physique from just one session per week: your body needs to be worked regularly and repetitively, with healthy eating patterns and relaxation included in the routine. So many 'healthy' children from the Western world are now purported to be overweight. You *can* make a difference through repetitive effort. I firmly believe that regular massage, physio and exercise routines at home will make a difference to any child, both physically and emotionally. There are, of course, quite severe degrees of cerebral palsy, which makes life even tougher for those children and their parents. But with determination, they too can make a difference to their child's development and quality of life.

Remember that each child is different
and should be encouraged to develop at
his or her own pace. Always encourage your child
to take the next step forward.

Pushing the boundaries

By almost three years of age, Callum could crawl independently and was quite a fast mover. (Most babies learn to crawl by six months of age and are walking by 12 months). I registered him at a preschool because both Brenda and I felt he needed the mental stimulation, since he couldn't walk. After assessing the situation at his playgroup on day one, Callum took control. He had a wonderful sense of humour and his speaking skills were above average. With his quite advanced communication skills, he managed to enlist the help of his classmates to do his fetching and carrying for him.

Callum also asserted himself in another way. Moving from class to class, he would grab a low wooden trolley with a handlebar that was filled with brightly coloured bricks and push it around with the teacher's books inside. Using the trolley for support, he felt empowered with his important duty for the teacher. This gave Callum a legitimate reason to be different from the other children without feeling disabled and less of a person. How lucky Callum was to have such good teachers who made every effort to integrate him into their class. Callum was the joker who loved to play tricks. This helped to establish a lovely atmosphere for Callum in the class.

When Callum progressed to walking with a tiny Zimmer frame when he was three, he was delighted to be able to move independently, laboriously lifting his feet in the special Spanish-made leather boots recommended by the hospital. Kids are tough, but my heart sank every time

Callum fell. I would pick him up casually and say, 'Upsadaisy! You're okay, darling', so as not to make a big issue out of it. It might have seemed harsh to onlookers, but with a little help Callum would just get back up and get on with the job of learning to walk. He had to be tough and accept things as they were.

Children do need some freedoms to encourage them to push their boundaries. It's just that much tougher when, the taller they grow, the harder they fall. Walking and balancing was difficult for Callum because he was tall. I was told to get him to walk 20 steps and then have him stand with his frame for 20 minutes. Twenty minutes is a long time for any child, never mind a child with weak muscles and a short concentration span. I devised a plan to make this exercise fun: I filled the bath to near full and placed lots of floating toys and foam shapes in the tub.

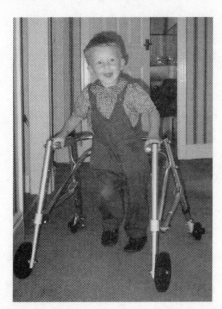

'Look at me, I can walk!'
Callum walking with his
Zimmer frame, aged three.

Callum had to race down the corridor to the bathroom and then stand against the bath, reaching in to retrieve the toys. It worked, and Callum loved this game.

In Australia, one mum, quite by chance, put a sticky note on her cerebral palsy son's good hand and was amazed to see him painstakingly reach across with his other hand to pull it off – helping him to learn to grasp, a skill he needed to learn. She turned this exercise into a game, and because her son enjoyed it, the repetition built up his muscles so that now he can use both hands.

Anything is possible, if you remain open and receptive to the universe's energy flow. Persistence is the key to success.

Two steps forward, one step back

Often Callum would make significant progress, becoming more flexible and falling over less often than before. Then, almost overnight, he would grow two-thirds of a centimetre and have to crawl out of bed because he was too stiff to walk. The falling over would start all over again. The exercise program would continue, but it was almost as if he had made no progress. The saying 'two steps forward and one step back' is so apt for children with cerebral palsy. It also applies to the one in eleven children who experience learning difficulties. Henry Ford had very little school education and still created an abundant life for himself. Richard Branson, the billionaire founder of the

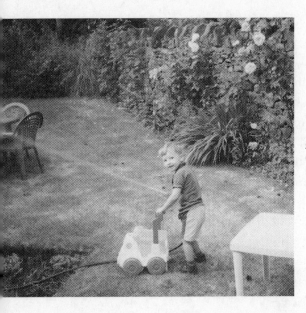

Callum watering the garden. 'If I hold it closer to my willy, will Mum think it's me watering the garden?'

Virgin empire, was told by his headmaster that with his lack of concentration and attention at school he would either wind up in prison or become a millionaire. He made his first million at 19 years of age from selling records. The rest is history. Every step forward, no matter how small, really does make a difference.

People would often see Callum holding onto my leg. If I had to move away, I either picked him up or sat him on the floor. It would have been easier to have left him sitting while I went about my chores, but it wouldn't have built up his muscle strength or his self-esteem. I would cajole Callum into helping me. He loved doing jobs with the understanding that he was 'helping' me and not doing his physiotherapy. As you can see from the photo of Callum watering the garden, he would grip tightly onto his plastic truck for balance.

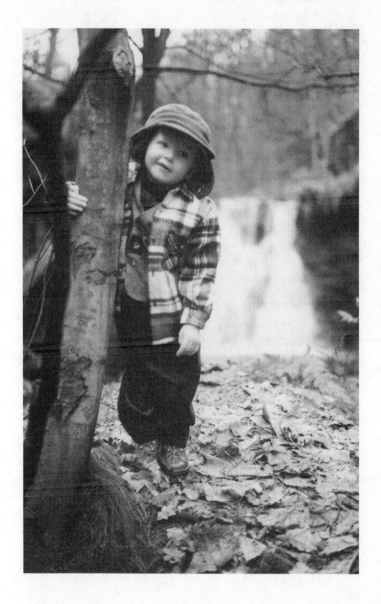

'Tree therapy'

There were times when I would ask a friend to act as a physical support for Callum. Callum would stand patiently, holding onto the friend's leg and not daring to move because of his balance. Suddenly the friend would move away or take a step, forgetting that Callum couldn't stand unaided. There'd be a loud thud as Callum hit the floor, then the friend would apologise, with Callum mumbling that it was okay and that he was fine. My poor friend would feel awful, but Callum and I understood that it was really okay!

Milestone upon milestone

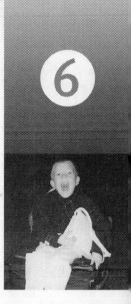

Small opportunities are often the beginning of great enterprises.

Demosthenes

MY MAJOR FOCUS during the period from 1994 to 2000 was Callum's wellbeing and working towards achieving the financial freedom to pay for the holidays that we looked forward to so much. Just months after Callum began physiotherapy and started to receive other medical support, I learnt that all parents of children with special needs in the United Kingdom can claim disability allowance from social welfare. This assistance is to help fund the special items or equipment that children with special needs require, as well as the necessary additional care. In Australia, permanent residents who have a child with special needs can apply at Centrelink for 'Carer Allowance'. There is so much support available – you just need to be aware of where to go for assistance (see pages 227–232 for a list of organisations to contact).

Both Callum and I needed regular breaks from the daily grind. With my work at the spa, hospital visits and the daily physio routine with Callum, as well as accounts work at night for my business, my good intentions for leading a balanced life often went out of the window. So I tried to get away every three months for a break with my son.

Occasionally, if there was a party or ball to go to, Callum would stay with the Owens family where his mates would keep him entertained while I enjoyed a night out with friends. Inevitably I would end up working longer hours, arrive late at the party and be the first to leave. My friends understood the situation, but it didn't give me many opportunities to meet a new partner. Still, everything in its time, I say.

In 1996 the strain of Callum's hospital visits, the divorce, financial worries and staffing problems at my spa began to take their toll. I had lost so much weight that I looked anorexic, and I had started to black out and fall, breaking my teeth. My body was covered in bruises.

That year I won a ski trip to Canada through the spa, and thought that the break would do me the world of good. While on the slopes, I blacked out and was taken to hospital. The doctors warned me that it was obvious I was very stressed, despite my joviality, and if I didn't slow down I would end up suffering a heart attack or a stroke in my early thirties. They certainly knew how to scare me into turning over a new leaf. I had the weight of the world on my shoulders and wasn't replacing the energy that I freely gave out each day. I had to learn to relax more and enjoy each moment.

On my return to England, I decided to sell my large health spa and work on my plan to franchise and open smaller spas that would be easier to manage. Within the month, the deal was done.

Despite our limited finances, every year Callum and I would invite all our friends over for our joint birthday celebration at home. We also made the most of inexpensive outings in our local area, such as the free open days at the local fire station.

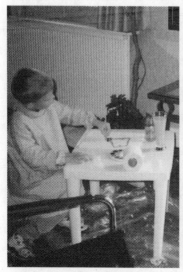 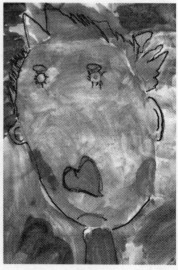

Callum painting, aged five – the next Van Gogh

Self-portrait, aged five – 'Gee, I'm handsome.'

To relieve my stress I'd spend evenings and weekends painting and designing. Callum and I found that we reallly enjoyed this creative time together.

It was at this time that my friend Suzanne suggested that I look into the Chinese art of feng shui, which is concerned with energy flow around the home and the placement of furniture and other objects to maximise health, wealth and wellbeing. I was hooked!

Every day we'd also put dance music on the stereo and dance in the living room. It helped me to stay positive, and it kept me fit – although I didn't have much problem there, due to lifting and carrying Callum whenever he got tired, which was often.

As my financial situation improved, I would take Callum to the driving range, and between us we would hit a basket of golf balls onto the range. Callum had all the jargon down pat: 'Mummy, you topped that one. Nice shot!' At two and a half he could 'play golf' if I held onto him while he took a swing at the ball.

Each passing year seemed to be marked by Callum's milestones and our celebratory holidays. The holidays we managed to take helped to break the monotony of our daily routine and were particularly encouraging for Callum, especially when at two years of age he learnt to snow ski. I would hire a sled so that I could transport him from the cabin to the slopes – as you can imagine, a wheelchair is hopeless in the snow! Other holidaymakers at the ski resort didn't know that there was anything wrong with Callum's legs when he was in the sled. We would then put on our skis and Callum would slide along under my legs. The hard ski boots and his natural snowplough stance gave him the support necessary to keep him on his tiny skis. He took enormous pleasure in telling everyone he could ski! It boosted his confidence enormously to know that he was learning to do what other children could, in spite of not being able to walk properly or see very well.

As you can imagine, travelling alone with Callum often wasn't easy. Travelling with any child or children is a challenge, but it can also be a joy. Callum would sit on the suitcases holding onto the skis while I battled to find trolleys and wheelchairs. I would be exhausted by the time we reached our destination, but the joy on Callum's face when he saw the mountains was worth all the effort. I could whiz off and ski for a few hours while Callum went to ski school or crèche with a group of children from all parts of the world.

To cover the expense of our holidays, which I considered a necessity to give us something to look forward to, I took on extra work. I was often working four jobs at a time: managing my health spas, doing freelance interior design work, writing freelance editorials for Condé Nast, and public speaking at conferences. I've always considered myself to be a fun-loving and expressive communicator, whether that is through the written word, my theatrical exuberance or the spoken word. I had been trained in South Africa by the Toastmasters Association to speak professionally, which gave me added confidence to talk on topics such as communication, sales and self-esteem to corporations, women's groups and universities, while my diploma in journalism gave me the edge to be able to submit travel and style articles, which I wrote after our exotic trips abroad.

From strength to strength

At the age of four Callum had had two years of eye patching and it had made a tremendous improvement to his vision. He could now see objects close to him, but his distance vision was still blurry. I had patched his eyes every day for up to seven hours since his eye surgery, so he was very used to this routine. He still couldn't walk unaided. The Airedale Hospital was still supplying Callum with special shoes and splints, and they also loaned me a MacLaren buggy, specially made for bigger children with walking difficulties, since most children outgrow their pushchairs between two-and-a-half and three years old. There was nothing bigger available other than a wheelchair, which could be quite depressing for a child aspiring to walk. The MacLaren buggy was lightweight and folded almost into a stick for ease of transportation for parents, unlike a wheelchair. But most importantly, it looked very much like the pushchair that Callum had just outgrown. Children do like to feel 'normal' and not so different from other children.

It was about this time that my mother showed Callum the *Forrest Gump* film on video, as mentioned earlier. He really loved the movie, especially the scene where Forrest attempts to run: his calipers miraculously spring off, and suddenly he is able to run like a normal boy. Callum was so inspired by this movie. He watched it over and over until the videotape wore thin. It was his greatest motivation. He could relate to the character of Forrest, and if Forrest could run, then so would he! One evening he told me it was his goal not just to walk but to run.

Callum was setting his own parameters and objectives.

He said he wanted to run like Forrest Gump more than anything in the world. I was so proud of him. Running was his motivation and desire. I would have been pleased just to see him walk, but I adjusted my goals to coincide with his. I promised him that when he took his first solo steps I would take him to Disneyland to buy some 'Lion King' running shoes.

Two weeks later Callum took his first independent steps. Callum had gradually developed walking skills by holding onto his wooden trolley at school, or his Zimmer frame. At first his balance was very precarious. But his desire to run took over, and brought out the courage to throw himself forward and attempt to move without support. He had many falls, but would pick himself up and mutter 'Oops!' and carry on. Like Thomas Edison, who undertook some 10 000 experiments before successfully inventing the electric light-bulb, Callum must have taken 10 000 or more attempts at walking and as many falls before his first two successful solo steps. Both the teachers and I cried.

> Our dreams and desires aren't the same
> as our children's. Our children have their
> own path to follow.

Naturally we visited Disneyland and bought the shoes. I worked 12-hour days and took on extra work to pay for the trip, working through the night from home as Callum slept so that I could still be a mama during the mornings and afternoons. At the age of 89, my

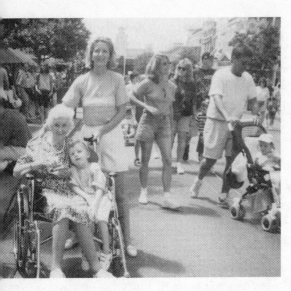

Shelley, Callum and Nanan at Disneyland. One wheelchair for two – cool!

grandmother accompanied us, so I pushed them both around Disneyland in an enormous wheelchair.

I was worn out, but very happy. It was a momentous occasion in Callum's life to be able to wear real running shoes. Nanan had always wanted to go to Disneyland, so it was a great adventure for us all. I was also achieving my goal to allow Callum to have the same worldly experiences he would have had if I had still been married and financially secure.

Ready for school

At age four and a half, specially fitted calipers were made for Callum to help him walk. At this time I was giving a lot of thought to Callum's schooling. Ruth McAlister, Callum's physiotherapist, suggested that he would be better off in a small class environment. If I could afford to send him to a private school, he would handle the smaller classroom situation better than he would a larger state school class. I preferred this to sending him to a special-needs school. If he needed a private school education, then that was what he would get!

Many of the private schools were very academically orientated. I wanted one that would be supportive of Callum's character and suit his personality, developing his strengths and assisting where he needed more support. Sally, one of the local mums who had similar requirements for her son, recommended Clevedon House School. The school had a swimming pool, which would help Callum's physical development, and a policy of only 12 children per class. It was ideal. The school gave permission for Callum to attend if he came out of nappies.

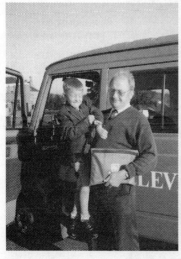
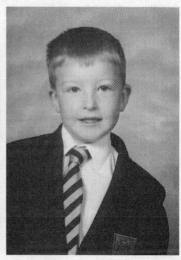

'What time do you call this, Mum?'   *School portrait, aged five*

This was all the incentive that Callum needed. We worked together as a team, mother and son. He loved the constant praise for his progress towards being nappy-free, and talked about his goal as if achieving it was inevitable. His bowels and intestines had strengthened over the years as we learnt what food his body could process. At the age of five Callum stopped wearing nappies.

What a momentous turning point this was in our lives. Callum's father agreed to pay the school fees in lieu of any maintenance or divorce settlement, which still hadn't been finalised. It was wonderful that Callum could go to a normal private school, with small classes, where he would be encouraged to reach his potential.

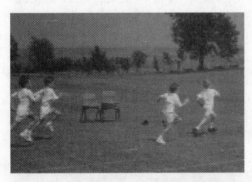

'Run, Callum, run!' Callum in the lead.

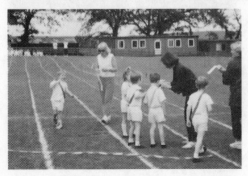

Callum finishing after the other competitors. It's not winning but participating that expands the soul.

Callum adored school. Of course he had several accidents, but the teachers seemed to handle these situations without making a big fuss. Callum had become very sensitive and embarrassed about his toileting, so their handling of the accidents was terrific. Callum blossomed in this environment, and the teachers allowed him to run in the school races and be just like the other children. His dream of running in a race, just like Forrest Gump, came true ... I was the most passionate mother there, cheering him to the finish line.

Callum attended his classmates' parties and we would invite his friends over to our place for sleepovers. Callum's friends would massage his legs and chase him around, or push him around the house in his wheelchair. One day we even invited the older boys over to pull the wallpaper off our walls! There were many laughs at our house that day. Inviting other children to our house would fill it with laughter and energy. Callum would also spend weekends at his cousins' and mates' houses so that he could experience how they lived.

Before long, Callum became a whiz on his computer. We ran our own toy sale, selling Callum's old toys, so that he could buy a Play Station. He also entered a dance competition and received a medal for his efforts. All of these activities and achievements boosted his confidence tenfold. It was so wonderful to see Callum's self-esteem go from strength to strength.

At the age of five and a half, Callum was still wearing eye patches, but he could finally see large marbles. By the age of six he could see hundreds and thousands on a cake. This was an amazing breakthrough. The Bradford Hospital orthoptists and I would hug one another at these milestones, and of course we hugged Callum too!

At school, after the initial day of getting to know one another, the children regarded Callum's eye patches and calipers as normal and almost didn't notice they were there until he fell over. Callum would always be sat at the front of the class to help with his vision, and the teachers and their support teachers made special time for Callum to complete his schoolwork and various projects.

Even today, Callum gets a lift to the sports field with the teachers and doesn't have to walk with the rest of the group. Callum developed an excellent memory in order to disguise his lack of good vision, which affected his reading skills. The teacher would read the words first and Callum would appear to read the words, but instead he was remembering what she had just said. Ninety-eight per cent of the time he would get away with this tactic, until he made a mistake by putting his own words or translation into effect. I often have to enlighten the teachers to Callum's clever ways of achieving results while disguising his lack of comprehension or ability to do the task the way the teacher intends. For example, Callum would learn his times and division tables sequentially, but if asked what is ten divided by two, he wouldn't understand how to do it because he had learnt the order of the tables by rote. He would be flummoxed and feel stupid, which would affect his class concentration and self-esteem. Yet his brilliant memory could regurgitate any information, so that when he was asked to repeat the two times table in order, he would do it with aplomb.

Many children find the linear learning method used by most schools difficult to grasp – it's best to find a way that suits each child. They may respond well to a visual method of learning, seeing the big picture first and then reducing it into its smaller components.

At Ruth McAlister's recommendation, Callum learnt to ride a horse when he was six. There were many horse-riding stables where we lived in Yorkshire. At our local stables, Carol, a woman specially trained in RDA (Riding Disabled Accreditation), was teaching children with special needs. All the stable hands were a delight.

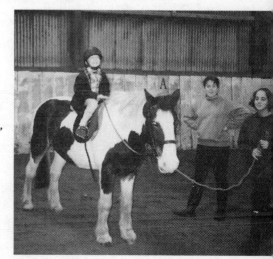

'It'll be polo next, Mum!'

Sometimes it was so cold waiting in the barn during the lesson that I joined the children's class, much to everyone's amusement. It was fantastic to learn to trot and jump, and Callum loved it because he could lead and was fast on a horse.

From four years old, he had pushed himself harder to walk unaided, and once he could do that he really wanted to play in the playground with the other boys, who would inevitably be kicking a football or chasing after a tennis ball in a game of catch. By seven, Callum could run and almost kick a ball in mid sprint without falling, even though his legs were long, thin and awkwardly turned in. His sheer tenacity kept him going. Callum's desire to be accepted as one of the boys kept him motivated, although many times the boys would get fed up with Callum missing, dropping or losing the ball, or at worst, falling over and making them feel guilty. He was always shown compassion when he most needed it. The girls were always there to mother him.

It reminds me of the story I was told by a friend about a dad and his son, who was mentally retarded. The boy had never achieved any form of success in anything practical, but he was loved and happy. The father was taking his son for a walk in the park when they came across two teams of youths playing a heated and obviously exciting game of baseball. It was the deciding game and the last team was batting. The little boy felt the excitement and was desperate to join in, and so the father asked if he could have a turn at batting. The pitcher scowled and looked at the boy, then glanced over at the opposing team's captain, who just shrugged back. You could see his brain ticking over … he thought and then smiled and said, 'Sure'. The two teams were confused and annoyed, but nobody said anything.

The excited boy grabbed the bat and the pitcher threw a gentle ball, hoping the boy would be able to make contact with his bat. He swung and missed, to no one's surprise, but on the second throw the boy struck the ball and the ball spun a few yards to the side. The bowler shouted 'Run, come on, run to first base – you can make it!' and then winked to the fielders.

The little boy ran as fast as he could. The fielder picked up the ball and purposefully threw it wide to miss the first post, so the boy made it safely. The whole team now twigged to what was going on and shouted, 'Run to second base!' and the boy ran for his life. Once again the ball was picked up, thrown wide and the boy was encouraged to keep on running. He made his first home run to the screams and shouts of glee from both sides. He had won the deciding game for his batting side.

Both teams had deliberately chosen to give this little chap the glory and make it happen for him. It certainly was an unforgettable day for the boy, his father and those passionate baseball players. No doubt the little boy's self-esteem, confidence and the desire to succeed in other things would have received an enormous boost from that experience.

Compassion can make a world of difference, even if it is just a kind smile.

Life for Callum and me was enjoyable because we made it that way. But it certainly wasn't all smooth sailing. On Callum's seventh birthday, he asked me if his dad didn't love him because he had wobbly legs. 'Of course not, darling,' I replied. 'Your dad loves you as much as he can in the best way he can.' My heart broke and I wondered how I could make it up to him.

Then he started watching a TV series featuring his favourite group at the time, 'S Club Seven'. One episode featured them singing to a little boy whose father had forgotten his birthday and not shown up for his party. Callum was mortified for the little boy.

Life can certainly be cruel. I learnt through the psychiatrists and psychologists at Airedale Hospital that you can't protect your children from harsh realities. When we went to see the first Harry Potter movie, Callum said that spending alternate weekends with his father made him feel like Harry Potter. I tried to make a joke that his dad never made him sleep under the stairs. 'No,' he replied, 'but I had to sleep on a mattress on the floor.' I know that isn't a real comparison, but I sat in the cinema in the dark with tears rolling down my cheeks. Callum just held my hand and whispered, 'It's all right, Mama. It just is. I'm fine about it. I have you. I love you.' My poor Callum. Not only has he had to contend with his disability, but he has also had to cope with his parents' divorce.

Fun and laughter are the best antidote.

By this time I had become a director of a TV production company through an association with some business networking groups. My reputation as a marketing strategist and my experience in the media world prompted a request by the board of directors of a local TV production company, RTV, to join their board as marketing director. My role was to attract advertisers and produce new programs. This opportunity enabled me to contribute positive programming and spread the word about health and wellbeing in a much more effective, visual and memorable way. I was given the flexibility to write, produce and present several programs, including 'Beautiful Babes' (to empower people's self-esteem, self-confidence and health), 'Posh People's Places' (to inspire people to strive to reach their goals and dreams), 'Broadly Yorkshire' (which highlighted the talents of people in the local area), and 'Kiddy Kapers' (in which Callum and his friends

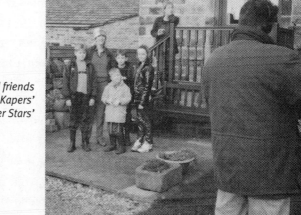

Callum, Shelley and friends on location for 'Kiddy Kapers' Super Stars'

starred). 'Kiddy Kapers' was produced to demonstrate the path to physical wellbeing through exercise. 'Art Attack' highlighted creative development and social conscience by taking children into hospitals and other disadvantaged sectors of the community.

In February 1999 I was given a copy of James Redfield's *The Celestine Prophecy*, an amazing tale of a spiritual journey. It awakened my desire to travel to South America, a continent I had learnt so much about when putting together tours while working in the travel industry in 1984. Coincidently, while I was reading *The Celestine Prophecy*, a brochure was posted through my door advertising a trip from Rio to Iguazu Falls, the Amazon, Machu Picchu, Lake Titi-caca and Leticia, Colombia. I just knew I had to take the trip.

I planned this adventure for Christmas, when Callum was to be at his father's for a week and then spend the rest of the holidays with my sister and his cousins. My friend Adele, who had heard me speak at a business network function and later befriended me, asked if she could join me on this journey of a lifetime, since it would be her first Christmas alone after her marriage split. Our South American journey turned out to be a life-changing experience, and so much fun.

Grab an opportunity when it jumps out at you,
even if you are not sure why or how.
The universe has a special way of giving you
what you need just at the right time.

On our first day in Rio, lying by the luxurious hotel pool, I sat for what seemed like an hour watching the most beautiful hummingbird sip nectar from a hibiscus flower. I was surprised by how small the bird was, yet how rapid its wing movements were. It brought to mind *The Celestine Prophecy*, in which the author describes people or animals joining 'synchronistically' with life, revealing their beauty. In my experience, the universe has a wonderful way of attracting exactly what you need once you have consciously decided what that is. 'Serendipity' and 'synchronicity' are my two favourite words. 'Serendipity' describes the fortuitous discovery of things you haven't sought for. 'Synchronicity' describes meaningful coincidences, when things start to happen in your life at just the right time. It's uncanny, but I have witnessed synchronicity over and over. The philosophy of *The Celestine Prophecy* basically states that we are all just vibrating molecules or another form of energy. The human spirit continues to grow, develop and experience a whole spectrum of feelings after death to eventually become one with the universe, almost like being a little part of God, experiencing the imperfect to appreciate what perfection really is. *The Celestine Prophecy* is a story of adventure, demonstrating how spiritually evolved beings keep stepping up to the next level of consciousness by following their intuition and creating their own realities. Many opportunities available to us are only seen by those who possess highly attuned values, such as faith, love, contribution and courage.

One example of synchronicity occurred at breakfast on Christmas Eve in the Amazon. My travelling companions asked me what outfit I was going to dress up in that evening, as I was renowned for my stylish image, whether I was in the city or the Brazilian jungle. As it was the festive season, I said that it would have to be my cream silk Marilyn Monroe dress with stilettos. I joked that if I had brought my tiara and wand I could have been the Christmas Fairy and made their Christmas wishes come true. I also told them that I hoped they would all make the effort to dress for dinner that night, and gave a knowing smile to our tour guide, Karen, who had confided to me that she wanted to start dressing up.

Our boat moored on the edge of the river, close to a leper colony. I didn't want to visit the colony to stare at the sick people, so I spent the day reading and lazing in the hammock on deck. That evening a hush came over the others as my heels clicked on the wooden floorboards on my way down to the restaurant. When I arrived they burst into laughter as Adele perched a pearl tiara on my head and handed me a wand! I couldn't believe it. They had wandered into a leper village in the middle of the Amazon, miles from anywhere, and in a little shack, among the handicrafts, they had found a gold wand, a tiara and a velvet dress for Karen!

By putting out your request to the universe, magic does happen. Somehow, just when you think of someone, they phone you or walk back into your life. This happens time and time again, so use your requests for the force for good.

That night I waved my wand and blessed all on board with their wishes and we danced and partied the night away.

On Christmas Day our group of ten exchanged the presents we had managed to purchase at a small Brazilian airport, and then went fishing for piranhas. Adele and I jokingly commented that at least in the Amazon we were saving our money, because there were no shops!

Later, to the beat of bongo drums, it was announced that Francesco Grippe, a local artist, had invited us to visit him as his privileged guests. His studio and residence were located in a wooden hut on stilts in the forest. As soon as I entered his studio, I saw the painting. I couldn't take my eyes away from the colours and beauty of the hummingbirds. I knew then that I had to buy it. I was already travelling with five suitcases (they don't call me 'princess' for nothing), so the 5 ft by 4 ft canvas was taken off its wooden frame and rolled up. The hummingbirds joined me on my journey. It was the perfect Christmas present to myself. So much for not shopping!

A week later, on New Year's Day in Peru, I found myself sitting on the mountain top at Machu Picchu. Adele had altitude sickness, and the best-looking doctor in Peru was looking after her. She was in heaven. All alone there I felt so energised. I found myself asking the universe what was my true path and what did I really want from life. The simple answer came immediately to mind. I wanted to live a more carefree, healthy life in Australia with Callum.

Yorkshire can be a particularly cold and wet place to live. Callum really suffered in the freezing winter months. His muscles would seize up, and in the mornings he'd have to crawl out of bed on his knees to make it to the toilet on time. Often he didn't get there quickly enough and he'd be so upset at having made a mess. Of course, I made light of the accidents, but it was awful to see him upset at the start of the day. I poured a lot of energy and effort into warming up his legs and cheering him up, washing floors, changing bedding, and doing his physio before going to work. It's hardly surprising that by the end of the day I was exhausted and often collapsed into bed shortly after Callum did. I had absolutely no energy left for a social life.

I knew that I had been putting my health at risk by working long hours and managing Callum on my own. I had achieved so much since my divorce, but it seemed that I had everything in life except time and romance. Callum was getting bigger and heavier. He wasn't bothered about holidays; he just wanted to spend more time with me, he said. How lucky I was to be loved unconditionally by this most courageous, beautiful and happy boy.

If we lived in a sunny climate, I reasoned, Callum would really benefit from the warmth by being more mobile and able to swim every day. It would help to develop his muscles. I had a strong desire to live in a place where I could look out of the window and see beautiful blue water every day, instead of working long hours to pay for our regular trips abroad. I wanted us to be able to spend more time outdoors and enjoy a more balanced life.

Ask and you shall receive. Meditation is one of the best ways of focusing on your inner desires and beliefs, and it revitalises your mind and body, giving you an energy boost.

We also needed to live somewhere where the medical services were first class. Callum's doctors agreed that this kind of lifestyle would be ideal for Callum. I longed to live in a place with a similar lifestyle and climate to South Africa, where I could continue to work on my speaking forums, TV shows, coaching, styling and writing. As a single person I would have returned to South Africa like a shot, but with the political situation there being so volatile and the crime rate so high, I didn't think it was a suitable place to raise my son.

I knew that for some years I had been a bit of a martyr, using Callum's medical condition as my excuse for remaining in England. I decided to take control of my destiny and apply for residency in Australia. If we were given the go-ahead, I would sell up, relocate and start a new life. If we didn't qualify, I would settle into life in the United Kingdom once and for all, franchise my salons, continue with my TV shows and write my book.

Decide what you want and go for it. Sometimes you don't know how and when, but the decision often attracts the outcome.

My ex-husband was quite happy for Callum and I to move to Australia, and he agreed in court that Callum would benefit from the move. So I applied to the Australian Embassy and put my business and house up for sale. Nothing stood in our way.

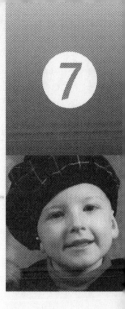

Straight and tall

*Exercise your imagination as you do
your body. The more you develop it,
the easier it will be to solve
problems and remember facts.*

Andrew Matthews

BY THE TIME Rory was seven, in 1999, I knew how to keep his legs and tendons elongated and supple despite his growth spurts, but I was increasingly concerned that his legs were still bent inwards at angles, hindering his ability to walk. Most of the time he was in the 'snow-plough position', great for his skiing, but not for his walking or balance.

An able-bodied child is able to stretch their muscles by walking and running, so that as their bones grow, so too do the muscles and tendons. However, the muscles of a child with cerebral palsy do not lengthen or stretch to keep pace with the lengthening bones. Instead, they contract and become fixed in rigid and awkward positions, especially in the legs. This muscle contraction can play havoc with the child's balance and cause loss of flexibility, although this can be overcome in time through hard work and physical therapy.

Surgery is one option that is considered when a child's movement is impeded by the contraction of muscles as the child grows. Surgeons are able to lengthen muscles and tendons that are too short. In the past, the only way to release the pressure on the tendons was to partially snip them, like a rubber band. However, this procedure could only be performed five times, otherwise the tendons would snap. Plus, lengthening the muscles weakened them, making it necessary for months of rehabilitation. Also, the surgeons need to determine exactly which muscles and tendons to lengthen, otherwise they risk making the problem worse.

In Callum's case, I never allowed the doctors to cut his tendons before he was eight years old, because I knew I could keep his tendons elongated and supple through his prolonged and repetitive physiotherapy program.

Another treatment option for muscle spasticity that enables children with cerebral palsy to walk more easily and have improved balance is botox injections. Botox, the Botulism toxin, which causes food poisoning, is also used in cosmetic surgery to reduce the appearance of wrinkles. As a treatment for muscle spasticity in children with cerebral palsy, the Botulinum Toxin Type A is dissolved in saline solution and injected into the muscles under either local or general anaesthetic. It has the effect of relaxing the muscles by blocking the signals between the nerves and the muscles, thereby reducing muscle stiffness. It acts on the muscles to enable them to grow more normally. Physiotherapy is still necessary with this treatment, and the injections need to be repeated at regular intervals to maintain the improvement in muscle tone.

It is important to note that these are not miracle cures for cerebral palsy. Botox injections can make the tendons too floppy if over-prescribed. I didn't want to take this risk with Callum. My instincts told me to steer away from both muscle-lengthening surgery and Botox injections. Yet now he was older, no amount of physio was making any difference to the way Callum walked or balanced.

Gait analysis

Then one day, quite by chance, I happened to see a TV documentary about gait analysis. Gait analysis combines the use of computers and video cameras to analyse a patient's walk. A camera records the patient walking, the patient's feet touch special force plates on the ground, and their leg muscle activity is recorded using a special recording technique known as electromyography. Doctors and surgeons are able to pick the abnormalities in the child's gait and ascertain whether they can improve walking patterns by means of physiotherapy or surgery. In 1999 it was an innovative method for monitoring leg and body movements electronically. It is still an ideal tool for athletes post-injury, or for children born with cerebral palsy.

I instinctively knew that it was exactly what Callum needed.

However, the paediatric surgeons we visited every three months didn't agree that it was necessary. My intuition was telling me otherwise. After a passionate plea to Callum's paediatrician, Kate Ward, she referred Callum to the Sheffield Children's Hospital, one of the largest hospitals in the United Kingdom and which had a Gait Laboratory. We waited 18 months for the appointment.

Finally Callum's appointment came around, and his leg and body movements were monitored accordingly. The special physiotherapists and the surgeons at Sheffield believed that Callum would indeed benefit from two major leg operations to straighten his legs. The surgery would allow him a much smoother gait or, in layman's terms,

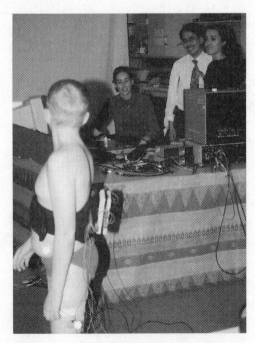

Callum wired up for gait analysis, just like an Olympic athlete.

enable him to walk tall and straight. I knew it! How lucky we were to have switched on the television at just the right time … it was serendipity, the universe working its magic once again.

With the marvellous techniques of gait analysis, the surgeons established that by rotating the muscles and fixing Callum's bones, he would have a much better chance of walking well, and perhaps even running. The analysis also suggested that no matter how much more physio Callum did, the inward rotation of his knees meant that his walk pattern could *only* improve by pinning his thighbones to his hips and turning the muscles.

The prospect of Callum undergoing two major operations was horrible, but Callum had no qualms. He wanted to have the surgery so that he could be tall and straight. He knew he'd be able to run faster, and that was his primary objective. I'll never forget the way Callum's face lit up when Mr Bell, the surgeon, asked what was his greatest wish. He boldly declared that his dream was to be tall and straight for our move to Australia.

The chances of Callum having surgery before we relocated to Australia were slim – there was an 18-month waiting list. I assumed that we'd return to England for the surgery, but at least we knew that the day would eventually come when Callum's legs would be straight.

I had hoped we would be in Australia for the start of the new millennium, but as that wasn't possible, I booked the next best thing – a trip to Antarctica! We organised an early Christmas celebration with the family in the United Kingdom, then we flew to South Africa. We spent time with my friend Amanda, and Callum enjoyed his first helicopter ride, over the Cape. From the air we were able to see our first whales, including a mother whale and her baby swimming up the coast.

From Cape Town we took a cruise to Rio, spent Christmas in Buenos Aires with my friend Joao, and then continued with the cruise to Antarctica, stopping off in the Falkland Islands and Uruguay on the way.

The crew was marvellous with Callum. He became one of them for the duration of the cruise, spending many days on deck with Captain Erik, or on stage in his tuxedo with the cruise director. He was allowed to skipper the boat and was given special ship privileges that the grown-ups didn't have. Since many of the guests were elderly, they took a shine to Callum, so I received a running commentary about the latest sighting of him on deck. It was a wonderfully relaxing holiday. However, being younger than most of the other passengers, I was expected to be the daring one, swimming in the volcanic waters of the Antarctic, starting off the dancing in Buenos Aires with the tango, and leading the fancy dress procession with Callum. It was enormous fun.

Antarctica was amazingly beautiful, with its glorious iceberg sculptures. You may be wondering how I got Callum onto the icebergs ... well, I am always the madwoman carrying a very big boy on her back, whether it is in a city centre when Callum has run out of energy, on the hills in the Falklands, or at the beach. There have been times when the weight of him has literally pulled the clothes off my back. On one occasion my flimsy dress-strap snapped and he had to hold onto it to keep my

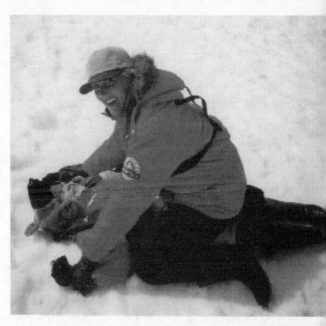

'Get off me, Mum! You're frightening the penguins.'

boobs from popping out as I struggled to hold onto him with my handbag slung around my neck. But the effort is always well worth it, just to see Callum's gorgeous smile. We returned from that holiday very content.

By this time I had received a couple of low offers for the house, but they were less than the sum of the mortgages. I couldn't afford to have negative equity. We had just received our visas for Australia, three of my staff running the health spas were pregnant and naturally wanting to reduce their hours, and one of my managers had been caught stealing and had been dismissed. The pressure was on for me to keep the business revenue high and liquidate my assets. Life became very hectic. I started to work long, erratic hours, once again dashing between the health spas. Fortunately, though, Callum had a marvellous babysitter, his close friend Mark, who would do all the 'boy' stuff with him, like woodwork and building.

Fate on our side

Magically, out of the blue we received a letter from the hospital offering Callum his operation in place of another child, who had fallen ill and couldn't undergo surgery. It was a dream come true for Callum. He was ecstatic! He was slotted in with just a week's notice. At nearly eight years of age, Callum was to have his legs straightened.

I distinctly recall the trepidation I felt for Callum in being admitted to Sheffield Hospital. There were so many children with injuries from accidents, child abuse or birth disabilities, who were far worse off than Callum: children with metal rods protruding from flesh and bone in order to elongate the child's legs; mothers with tales of using 230 cotton buds per day to clean the open wounds. Brave, brave children and their parents.

Callum and I had brought along a 6 kilogram supply of 'magic' jellybeans. Needless to say, they disappeared very quickly, gobbled up by the many children to ease the pain of any injections or foul-tasting medication. Word soon spread through the children's wards that Callum's mum was a glass-slipper-wearing princess (in fact, they were diamante-studded perspex mules) with magic powers, and different coloured eyes! The nurses scurried back and forth for handfuls of jellybeans as the news filtered around that the magic sweets made wishes come true and took away much of the pain.

The power of magic for children is amazing. To see their little eyes widen and their faces smiling is priceless.

The nurses made up a camp bed for me next to Callum's bed on the eve of his surgery. I told mysterious stories to the children in the ward until their medication kicked in and they fell asleep. The next morning the doctors were on their rounds when the dishevelled 'princess' made a run for the bathroom to change before Callum was wheeled down to surgery. He had a huge grin on his face – he couldn't wait to have straight legs. Before long he was sleeping like a baby, and the nurses ushered me out of theatre.

My head was spinning and I felt sick. I ran past the clown and Disney motifs on the walls, which seemed to be closing in on me. I couldn't get out of the hospital quickly enough.

Fresh air at last! I walked across to the park opposite the hospital and perched on a bench with a view of the lawns and flowerbeds. It was a very peaceful spot, but my heart was racing, my head was throbbing and tears were streaming down my cheeks. At that moment I really could have done with a bear hug.

Two hours later it began to rain, which I welcomed because no one could see my tears.

After three hours the sun re-emerged and steam started to rise off me!

After four hours the university students began to stroll across the lawns, some holding hands and laughing, others deep in serious conversation, and others immersed in their own thoughts. I felt very alone.

Was it time yet to return to the hospital?

I went back to the ward and waited to be called down to the recovery room. Finally ... Callum was ready. In the recovery room I went over to see another young boy just waking from the haze of surgery. I wasn't his mummy, but I held his hand and congratulated him on his bravery until she arrived. Why was it taking so long for Callum?

Then there he was, my angel-faced boy, the 'Lion King', so called because of his golden mane of hair. He smiled dreamily and asked, 'Are my legs straight, Mum?' I looked under his blanket but I couldn't tell because of the casts.

'Yes, perfectly,' I replied, with fingers crossed.

> It isn't easy to watch your child go through the trauma of surgery, but it is worth it to see the results of all our efforts, love and concern.

Those next few days were awful to watch. Callum vomited frequently from the anaesthetic and was kept on an epidural drip for several days to relieve his pain. And of course there was a catheter for his bladder. He had long blue casts from his toes to his thighs, with a bar stretching from ankle to ankle to keep his legs apart. Callum loved those long blue casts. They meant victory! My mother made him some special shorts with Velcro on each side because the bar between his ankles prevented any other type of clothing being put on.

In the hospital the physiotherapist taught me how to lift Callum into a wheelchair, onto his commode and

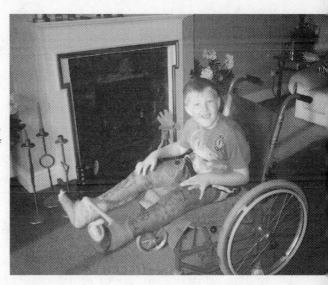

*Callum proudly
showing off
his casts*

onto his back to strengthen his stomach and lower back
muscles and tendons prior to the ambulance ride home.
My car had been smashed up outside the hospital the
night before and had had to be towed away. Had these
vandals no idea? If they were to spend a day in the
children's wards helping to care for the sick children
they might appreciate that there are people much worse
off than themselves. Maybe then they would never want
to commit such destructive acts again. At least it broke
the monotony of hospital talk, and the sick children
thought it was terrible but adventurous at the same
time. What irony!

Due to the tendon release between Callum's hip
bones and thighs, his natural reaction after the surgery
was to curl up, which would then cause him pain when
straightening, so it was important to get the flexibility
into those tendons as soon as possible after surgery by

turning Callum onto his stomach from the sitting position and pulling his tendons in the opposite direction. Every movement hurt him and he cried, but he would also smile when he saw my despair. 'It's all right, Mum. It'll be worth it!' What a brave boy.

I had to ensure that I ate well and looked after myself in order to be able to lift him. The doctors and surgeons advised that Callum's rehabilitation would take 12 months. Looking back, I don't know how we coped for all that time.

The recuperation period revealed to me reserves of energy and stamina I never knew I possessed. Pushing Callum and his heavy casts in a wheelchair, lifting him in and out of my two-seater sports car, with a wheelchair poking out of the back (we had to leave the roof down, even in the rain), and carrying him over my shoulder while I gripped the stair rail up to our front door, certainly took its toll. Despite being a highly energised person, I was often exhausted and accident-prone. I know that many of you must be thinking that I am a crazy, impractical and possibly selfish woman to drive a sports car, but I do believe we should remain true to ourselves. I have always been passionate about cars. Why shouldn't I still have the pleasure and allow my child the thrill of riding in a sports car? The mountain climber who becomes an amputee doesn't have to stop climbing because he has lost his leg.

Where there is a will, there is a way.

If prosthetics allow him to climb, then he can continue to follow his dream and live with passion. Erik Weihenmayer, a 32-year-old blind man, is currently attempting to climb Mt Everest with Baba Munundra Pal, a team-leader who has one leg. In 1998, Tom Whittacker, an American with an artificial leg, succeeded in climbing the 8850-metre-high mountain in Nepal. These are people living with passion in spite of the odds.

An acceptable offer had by this stage been made on the house, but fortunately, the sale fell through and we were able to continue living in our one-level home. Callum was delighted too because he didn't have to go to school during this time. He had lost a lot of confidence in the previous two terms because the new headmaster didn't seem to like his personality.

Rachel Dennison, Callum's devoted support teacher, was an angel. She missed teaching Callum, so she offered to teach him at home during the day so that I could return to work. After several months, Callum's casts were removed with an electric saw. It was the first time Callum

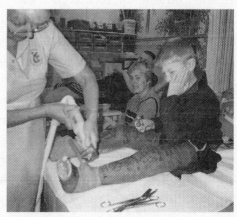

'Oh boy, that saw is scary!' Callum having his casts removed in hospital.

127

lost it completely. He screamed the place down, mainly in fear of the saw. The six scars looked horrendous. His casts were replaced by leg splints, covered by material. Callum then underwent home physiotherapy with Stephan from Airedale Hospital. He had to re-learn how to walk. Rachel helped with Callum's care routine as well as providing his schooling needs for the first six months after surgery. She taught him all about Australia and fed him up, too, with her home-cooked meals. Callum certainly enjoyed her cooking and teaching, and I owe much to Rachel and her family for lovingly supporting us both when I was in the midst of selling the businesses, the house and doing all the necessary tasks before our relocation to Australia.

This was to be our last Christmas in England, and it was Callum's father's turn to have him for Christmas. I thought it would be nice for both of them to spend that extra time together. However, at Christmas Callum's father announced that his plans had changed – Callum couldn't visit him for the holidays as planned. Callum said he wasn't bothered, but truly he was crushed. I knew it when he announced that he hated Christmas and he no longer believed in Santa. At the last minute, I rearranged my work plans and booked a flight for us to travel to Lapland – yet another trip paid for on my credit card. The universe would somehow have to provide me with more wealth to pay for it! Callum needed some magic in his life, and even I returned from Santa's village believing that Santa really exists!

Of course the wheelchair was hopeless in the snow. I looked like I was trying to breakdance and somersault in one direction as the wheelchair skidded and glided

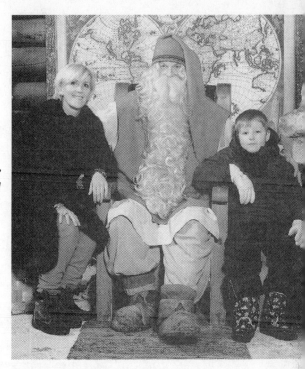

Shelley, the 'real' Santa Claus and Callum, Lapland.

in the other. We solved the problem by hiring a sled so that Callum could be pulled around on the snow, and he also enjoyed reindeer and husky-dog sled rides, Skidoo racing over the frozen rivers and drilling holes in the ice to fish.

Callum was a big hit with the other children at the hotel. He made good friends with Milo, who wanted to know what Callum's middle name was, and why. I explained that I had chosen 'Callum' if he was blond and 'Rory' if he was red-haired. 'But he has red hair!' Milo protested. So I explained that Callum's father preferred the name Callum and I liked both names, so he had become Callum. Well, that was it. It became a game for the boys. They both insisted on

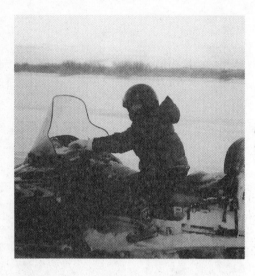

007 on a Skidoo in Lapland

being called by their middle names for the duration of the holiday, which was tricky to remember after eight years of calling him 'Callum', but after many laughs and quite a few 'C-rory's, I got into the swing of it.

On our return to the United Kingdom, Callum started a new school in our village. The first day when I picked him up from school I asked for 'Callum' and nobody knew who I was talking about! From that time on, Callum insisted that he wanted to be called Rory. As far as he was concerned, 'Callum' was what he was called when he was a disabled boy and 'Rory' was his new name, the new him with straight legs. What could I say but 'Okay, Rory!' It was *his* life and *his* name, after all. He knew his own mind and I was proud of him, besides which he is definitely a Rory redhead. The children and teachers at his new school were lovely, and they marvelled at Rory's ability to get about in his wheelchair, and later on his crutches.

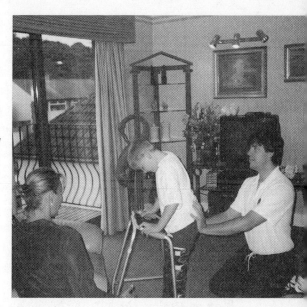

Callum with Rachel and
his physiotherapist,
Stephen.

It took nearly a year of hard work, a lot of 'bullying' from his physio Stephen, and daily exercises, for Rory to be able to move again from a wheelchair to a Zimmer frame and then on to crutches.

It was soon Easter. A couple had expressed interest in buying the house, and some business investors had come forward for my health spas. With so many projects on the go, combined with working long hours, managing Rory's physio and taking him to his hospital appointments, I had had very little time for pleasure in the previous 12 months. It was time for us to have a change of environment and get some fresh air.

My friends from Switzerland, Jenny and Martin, were spending Easter in Nairn, Scotland, so I decided to meet up with them and visit the castles of Scotland with Rory before we were to leave the United Kingdom for our new

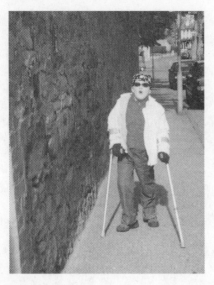

Long John Silver minus the parrot. Rory walking with crutches in St Andrews, Scotland.

life in Australia. On our journey through what the locals call 'God's country', we visited no less than 48 castles!

While in St Andrews I met a lovely gentleman whose daughter had been born with cerebral palsy and was still in a wheelchair. He was aware that Rory had cerebral palsy, and was amazed to learn that he had also been born blind and yet was doing so well. He had never heard of gait analysis, or many other treatments that I mentioned. As he related his own family's story, it became apparent that his wife had effectively martyred herself by never leaving her daughter in anyone else's care. He had lovingly stood by his wife and daughter, but they had no social life outside of work. They hadn't taken a holiday for 20 years, nor gone out for dinner to a restaurant or stayed with relatives. It was such a sad story, and to me it sounded like a very unhealthy situation for all of them, not just for the parents. Their daughter had not been

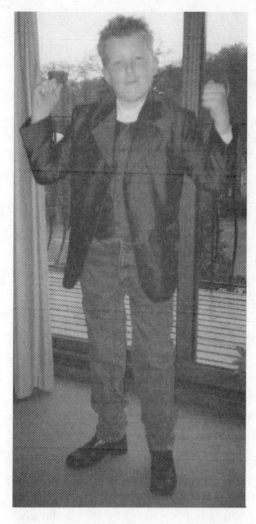

Straight legs – 'Yahoo!'

given the opportunity to develop independence or to grow spiritually or mentally. They were obviously devoted to her, but to an unhealthy degree.

This gave me a real incentive to work towards completing my book and getting it published, so that it

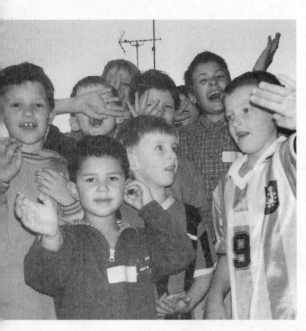

'Bye, Rory – we'll miss you!'

might help those people who were quietly battling on in the only way they felt was possible.

By the end of that year, Rory had lovely straight legs, although he walked with an obvious limp. I was so proud of him. He had already gone through so much in his life. He just wanted to be loved and accepted and to be the best person he could be. In the past year he had endured a great deal of pain, discomfort and the humiliation of being totally reliant on others for his toileting and bathing. He had re-learnt how to stand up and walk, and now he could almost run again. Rory was ready for take-off. He had no qualms about leaving England. As one door closes, another opens.

Australia, here we come!

Hello, Australia!

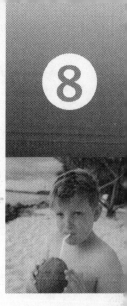

We are all in the right place at the right time for our lessons in life.

RORY RELISHED EVERY MINUTE of our move to Australia, from watching the professional packers load our car and our goods onto the container, to our trip to the other side of the world via Las Vegas, the Grand Canyon, San Francisco and Fiji.

Weighing up what each major city in Australia had to offer, I had decided that Sydney, despite its expensive real estate, had everything we were looking for. To me it is one of the prettiest cities in the world, with its beautiful harbour, cosmopolitan lifestyle, major television networks and every kind of leisure activity imaginable – from glamorous racing at Royal Randwick and concerts at the

Opera House, to beach volleyball and surfing. What more could we possibly want?

One month after departing England, we arrived at Mascot Airport in Sydney, not knowing a soul. Our stop-overs had left us relaxed and tanned and ready for the challenge of starting a new life. Our bags had been damaged in the trip over, so while we sorted things out the Qantas employee at the desk chatted with us, commenting on Rory's walking. She explained that her nephew had cerebral palsy and urged me to write a book about Rory's experiences and send her a copy. I had the overwhelming feeling that we were in the right place at the right time, a feeling that has stayed with me since we arrived in Australia.

A hotel in Potts Point became our home for six weeks until we found the right property to rent. From our hotel room we enjoyed spectacular city skyline and harbour views. At night the whole city twinkled with silvery, red and blue neon lights. We were in a prime vantage point for some impressive firework displays during our stay at the hotel.

Rory and I spent our days sightseeing and checking out the home rental market in the Eastern Suburbs. We were thrilled with the sights but became disillusioned with what was available in the housing market. However, we did love the $3 million-plus pads on the waterfront! We were typical 'Poms', with inflated ideas of what we could buy with our money.

Rory gave up looking with me after the twentieth house inspection. Eventually I found an apartment that fulfilled our criteria: water views, a swimming pool and a good school within walking distance. But then I was informed by the shipping agents that our container-load of belongings had arrived, with many of the contents damaged due to poor packing, despite having paid for the job to be done professionally. Quarantine and customs officials were delaying the release of our container. Unfortunately this delay led to the apartment being offered to someone else.

At about the fiftieth home inspection I pulled up at the kerb and knew instantly from the exterior that there was no point in inspecting the house. I got out of the car and began to apologise to the blonde woman standing on the footpath, who I presumed was the agent, saying, 'Thanks, but no thanks.' In fact she was a *Sydney Morning Herald* property reporter by the name of Cindy. She asked me where I would be looking next. 'Cape Cabarita! My agent assures me I'll love it.'

'You will,' she replied, and sure enough, the next apartment was everything we were looking for: it was modern, had a pool and views of the water, and there was a lovely school nearby. It was perfect.

Home sweet home

I hadn't planned on apartment living, but this one was luxurious. It had new cream carpets, a new kitchen and bathrooms, a lock-up garage and was surrounded by landscaped gardens with gardenias, jasmine and lavender, a clean pool, gym, tennis courts and a jacuzzi. Best of all, I didn't have to worry about cleaning or maintaining any of the gardens or communal facilities!

Our car and furniture were still being held up by customs, and the insurance company had sent out a loss

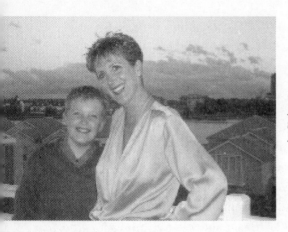

'Home is our paradise.' Shelley and Rory on the balcony of their Sydney apartment.

assessor. I didn't want to risk missing out on another apartment, so I signed the lease, paid the bond and ordered new whitegoods.

Finally I could relax and focus on my work. I had a new TV show reel produced with the Sydney Opera House as my backdrop in order to market myself to casting agents. I submitted my book to several publishers in Australia and the United Kingdom, and sent my TV script for a program I had written called 'Beauty and the Feast' to TV producers.

Another week passed and the furniture still hadn't arrived, but Rory's new school was starting classes again after a break. So we moved into the empty apartment on the eve of his first day at school, with just our cases of clothes and my laptop.

We had been happily surprised by how hot and sunny the July days in Sydney were, but the winter nights were chilly. The first night in our new apartment was so cold that we had to wear many layers of clothes to keep warm. We looked like the Wombles of Wimbledon Common, but at least we could laugh about it!

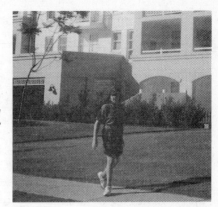

Rory walking to school in Sydney on his first day. 'Now I've done it, can I have a lift, Mum?'

On his first day at an Australian school, Rory was very excited. Significantly, Rory walked to his new school. Yes, *walked*. With butterflies in my stomach and feeling very anxious for him, I busied myself with my show reel and managed to buy a gas fire and sleeping bags for our second night in our beautiful, barren apartment. We were enjoying the novelty of being able to sleep in a different room each night and visualise where our furniture would go.

Rory's first day at school was super. His teacher, Mrs Claro, was the head of computers, Rory's favourite subject, and his classmates were lovely with him, especially after hearing his story of the car accident and seeing the scars on his legs. It was such a relief for me. That night, despite the fact that it was the middle of winter, Rory and I swam in the pool and sat in the hot jacuzzi in the dark, happy to gaze at the stars and reflect on how lucky we were.

> Gratitude is one of the most uplifting feelings. It keeps you focused on all the positive things in life.

With still no sign of our furniture, our first birthday in Australia, in July 2001, was the quietest birthday we had ever had. I was on a property developer's course, and although all 200 people at the seminar wished me a happy birthday, there was no big party this time, and Rory celebrated with his two new friends, James and Laura. Rory, however, was delighted with his new treat, a DVD player.

At last our furniture arrived – all 272 boxes! My car had been bumped and banged during transit because the packers had forgotten to secure a crate around it, so I sent it off to the garage for repairs and concentrated on the daunting task of unpacking the boxes. It took me 14 hours a day over seven days. I was physically drained, as the chemicals sprayed on the boxes during quarantine gave me severe nosebleeds. By the end of the week my back and hands were so sore that I would flinch at the slightest knock. The furniture that wasn't damaged suited the apartment perfectly. With paintings and sculptures collected from my travels around the world, our apartment became the warm and welcoming home we had both visualised. We celebrated our house-warming party with a picnic on the lawns of Cape Cabarita while watching and listening to a jazz band, then followed the picnic with dessert back at our apartment.

Soon after we moved in, a drama unfolded. I had arranged to meet with one of the Channel 7 TV executives, and wanting to look my best, I booked an appointment at one of my favourite international hair salons. Unfortunately the colourist left the chemicals on my hair a little too long and my scalp was burnt. My hair colour was no longer blonde – it had turned almost grey with pink roots! After seven hours in the salon, I left with dark, frazzled hair, missing in tufts. I cried all the way home.

How could I go for my interview with the TV executive? I no longer resembled the person in my show reel or professional photographs. My hair was dropping out in handfuls and it looked as if a dead animal was perched on my head. I was mortified. Another stylist evaluated my hair, and suggested I took photos. But there was nothing they could do as my scalp and hair were truly burnt. The only solution was to wait for my hair to grow back. I postponed the meeting with the TV executive until I had bought a wig.

For the next five months I wore a hat or a wig. I felt so low, and I became a virtual recluse. I developed fainting spells and all the symptoms of stress: panic attacks, heart palpitations and weepiness. I didn't seem to be able to control my emotions.

Breaking my shell

I withdrew from life, but I still went through the motions for Rory. One day at our pool I met Corrine and her two little boys, one of whom, Andrew, had cerebral palsy, which mainly affected his speech. Corrine had worked hard to help Andrew with physio, massage and alternative therapies. I showed her how to improve his speech by talking on his arm, as I had done with Rory. Andrew and Rory clicked right away and became best friends. Rory would demonstrate to Andrew some of the things he had learnt to do, and Andrew would hold Rory's hand to balance him.

Again I felt there was a purpose to my mishap. Perhaps I just needed to relax, trust the universe and stop trying to make things happen too quickly? Pacing the house at five in the morning, I switched on the TV to see an infomercial for personal development. 'Do you need inspiration?' Yes. 'Do you need new hope?' Yes ... yes ... yes. I bought into the Anthony Robbins program.

> It is said that the teacher appears when the student is ready. It is all down to timing.

I voraciously read inspirational books and plugged myself into motivational tapes. I really felt the need for mentoring during this trying time. It was spooky, because in England I had often been described as the female version of the American Anthony Robbins, but had never known who he was, and here I was in Australia, his new student and fan.

Corrine and I would take our morning walk around the bay together. It certainly lifted my spirits to see the jumping fish, the parrots and pelicans, as well as the beautiful boats bobbing on the water, and the distant city skyline. Despite my hair trauma and missing out on work with the TV studios, I was still very glad to be in Sydney.

We had already made some wonderful friends in our new homeland, friends who insisted that Rory and I shouldn't be alone for our first Australian Christmas. We enjoyed a lavish seafood barbecue with Corrine and her family and then went on to our friend Tina's place for a grand Christmas barbecue. It was a gorgeous day: Rory heaved with laughter and I was very glad of the company, although I still felt a little subdued in the company of others.

On Boxing Day we headed to a farm in Gunnedah, a country town north-west of Sydney. Naively, I thought the trip would only take two to three hours. Eight hours later we arrived at Jonathan and Rebecca's farm! It was a wonderful surprise to discover that the farm was on vast acres of land: the 'pond' we had heard about was really a lake, and the 'hills' surrounding the farm were mountains.

Just as we had seen in so many Australian films, there were wild kangaroos bounding across the paddocks and lazy, fat koalas hugging the trees. It was a genuine outback experience. Jonathan and Rebecca had laid on a sumptuous Christmas feast for us. Over the next few days Rory busied himself finding junk metal scraps from old tractors and welding them together to create sculptures.

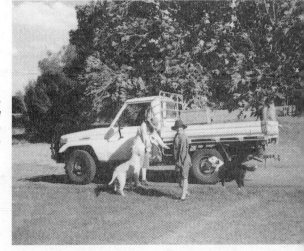

'Are you sure you're a Pom?' Rory and Rebecca on the farm in Gunnedah

143

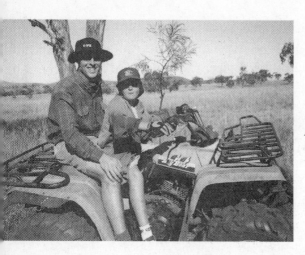

'Who needs to run
when you can ride?'
Jonathan and Rory
on the quad bike
in Gunnedah

He also went quad biking (a bike with four wheels for use over rough terrain) and drove a tractor fitted with satellite navigation to ensure that fields are ploughed in a straight line. He was in his element.

On New Year's Eve, back in Sydney, we attended a masquerade dinner dance. I was still very conscious of my hair, but the temptation to spend the evening with friends, watching the spectacular firework display above the Sydney skyline, was too great to resist. My English neighbours Gill and Pete accompanied us, while their lovely daughter Jamie babysat Rory. I felt immense joy that we were starting a new year settled in this heart-warming and friendly country.

Focusing on the positive brings joy
to your heart, no matter what
life throws at you.

February soon arrived and one of my best friends, Lorraine, arrived from London. It was so lovely to share our new home with a friend from our former life. I was sad when Lorraine left, but we had our trip back to the United Kingdom to look forward to eight weeks later.

In April 2002 we stopped over in Bali and Bangkok on our way to England. In Bangkok we shopped and visited the temple sights. Because of the heat, we spent our afternoons lazing by the pool. One day we noticed a young man on crutches taking very slow, laborious steps to reach our side of the pool. His family pushed the wheelchair around and made themselves comfortable on the sun beds. Twenty minutes later, the young man on crutches made it around too. It took him great effort, determination and energy. He could have had an easy ride, but his determination to learn how to walk again after suffering a serious head injury carried him forward – one step at a time.

We applauded his efforts. It was like seeing a bigger version of Rory struggling to make progress. The young man's name was Stuart, and his face lit up at our applause. He was amazed to learn that Rory was once like him – on crutches and having to re-train his legs to walk. Rory was very eager to show Stuart how he could swim too, and a new friendship blossomed. The incredible coincidence we soon discovered was that Stuart lives in Gunnedah, on the farm right next door to that of Jonathan and Rebecca, with whom we'd spent Christmas. Was this synchronicity working its magic once again?

Back in the United Kingdom

Our holiday in the United Kingdom was a whirl of meetings with Rory's doctors and surgeons, and spending time with family and friends. Rory spent two days with his father, which was the first time Rory had seen him since we left England and the first time Rory and I had been apart for ten months. He ran back into my arms after his brief visit.

Rory and I flew from England to see my mother in her new house in Spain, where she had moved to be near friends and enjoy sunnier climes during her retirement. The time with Mum was very meaningful to us – a time to talk, reflect and share our feelings honestly. One night we chattered until the early hours of the morning, airing feelings that needed to be aired. It was very cathartic for me. In the past I had avoided confrontation and kept quiet for the sake of peace, rather than being open and true to my spirit. This was the first time that I could explain to Mum how much I loved her and that while I was raising Rory I had had to keep my distance because I often felt criticised. Mum was great about it all. She acknowledged that it used to upset her to watch me doing physio on Rory. She also acknowledged that if she had had to care for him she would not have done the repetitive exercises, and he would still have been in his wheelchair.

It was so good to hear her approval, although by now I had grown spiritually to the point where I no longer really needed approval. It was so cool. Mum said that her criticism of me had stemmed from her concerns about my health and wellbeing, living on adrenaline alone, but she was proud that I had followed my heart and my intuition, because she could now see how much Rory and I had achieved both physically and emotionally. It seemed to me that Mum had also come a long way. Relinquishing the strings attached to your children is one of the hardest things to do. She was still finding it hard, especially with my sister, who had remained her focus while I had sought my independence. As Kahlil Gibran says:

> Children are of the parent,
> but do not belong to the parent:
> it is their job to send them out into
> the world to live and experience.

Back in Sydney, our birthday celebrations one year on were very different from the previous year's. Rory had a house full of friends in fancy dress, and he declared it his best party ever! I took my first helicopter-flying lesson and later celebrated with friends by having drinks at the Sydney Opera House, followed by Latin dancing at the Rocks. In just one year in Sydney we had achieved so much, simply by giving openly of ourselves and by having faith that life would unfold as it should.

Just when life was going so smoothly, I was involved in a car accident. Once again an unfortunate incident became a blessing. I met an inspirational physiotherapist, Natalie Simon, who shares my vision to open a health sanctuary. We are now working on my project together.

The accident also helped to renew my appreciation for how precious life is and how important relationships are. My lovely friends Brie, Gail, Sue, Maggie and Marie came to my rescue over the weeks of rehabilitation from whiplash by generously lending me cars or chauffeuring me to physiotherapy sessions and charity meetings that I would have missed without their kindness.

Christmas 2002 came around so quickly. We spent our second Christmas Day in Australia on Whale Beach with our friends Tina and Andy and their two children, enjoying the sunshine and festive atmosphere. New Year's Eve was also special, as Rory and I watched the Sydney fireworks from Cremorne Point with our friend Dermot Reeve, the English cricketer, and his family.

After Christmas, an unscheduled cruise around Australia was advertised. The ship had been scheduled to cruise to Bali, but due to the bombings in Bali, the itinerary was changed to include a leg around Australia. We decided to book the trip. Synchronistically, Captain Erik (from our Antarctica cruise) docked his ship in Sydney Harbour. We embarked on our Australian cruise, visiting Brisbane, Hamilton Island, Cairns, the Great Barrier Reef, Thursday Island, Darwin, Kakadu, Broome and Perth. What a beautiful country Australia is. Rory loved every minute of the cruise, much of which he spent on the bridge with the captain or in the kitchens with the chefs. I teamed up with a lovely family from Sydney and a group of English tourists, laughing the days away and spending the evenings dancing – it was perfect.

In February 2003 we hosted our dear friends from Switzerland, Jenny and Martin, showing them the picturesque sights of New South Wales. Hot on their heels arrived my most loyal and supportive friends, Jacquie and Julian, from the United Kingdom. How uplifting it is to be able to share our new life with friends from different parts of the world.

Today, Rory can see with average vision. He has long, straight legs, with scars and bruises as proof of his efforts to walk. He attends a public school that he can walk to independently. His school friends come over to play, and the other mums often help out with pick-ups and after-school invites. He has performed at the Sydney Opera House in a musical – *Singing in the Rain* – as the truncheon-swinging policeman. He plays handball like the other kids, swims like a fish, and now lives the life of an able-bodied boy. And with his new Australian 'twang' he sounds like a mini Rolf Harris! He is a miracle on straight legs.

In March 2003 Rory had another operation, this time on his foot. It was performed by a dedicated team of surgeons at the Sydney Children's Hospital, led by Dr Michael Stenning, and the aim of the surgery was to perfect Rory's gait and remove his slight limp. After the rehabilitation, no one will ever know that he once had problems walking.

Rory has been invited to visit the United States in July 2003 to share his story of courage with the children at Anthony Robbins's Discovery Camp. Rory's speech begins with the words:

'I am Rory Sykes. I was born blind, and ten years ago my mother was told I might never walk. I am a miracle

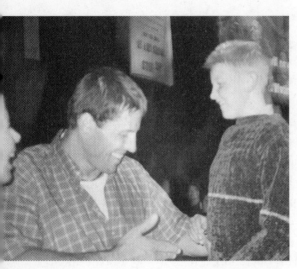

Anthony Robbins shaking hands with Rory. 'You're my hero, Tony. Want to marry my mum if I marry your wife?'

on legs; Anthony Robbins even said so. I am proof that miracles do happen. I am proof that the past does not equal the future. It isn't what happens to you in life that counts, it's what you do about it that matters ...'

My desire was always to see Rory live a normal, happy life and be able to travel the world like any other boy, so my dreams have been realised.

I have established a role on the TV program 'Beauty and the Beast', a panel chat show with six wonderful women and the witty Doug Mulray as host. I have signed up with an agent for acting, professional speaking and voice-over work. My speaking career in Australia has begun to flourish and I have joined the committees of three wonderful associations, the Australian National Speakers Association, Australian Spirit in Business and BaySports Association. I am have joined the board of directors for Anthony Robbins's charity, Magic Moments, as well as formed the 2B1 Foundation in readiness for establishing a charitable health sanctuary for children and their parents. This has given me the opportunity to meet some wonderful, spiritually aware people, who are helping me to achieve my goal of raising finance for my own TV project, a lifestyle program highlighting all aspects of image and wellbeing, and for the 2B1 sanctuary.

Rory and I truly hope that sharing our story with you has inspired you to believe that you too can make a difference in your life and in the lives of your beautiful children. Follow your heart, trust your intuition and live with passion.

Parents

*Close your eyes and listen to the surrounding echoes of
   mortality*
*Hear your heartbeat, entrap the energy, and solve the
   mysteries of humanity.*
Float in the beauty of your child's first smile,
Dance to the beat of your child's style.
Embrace the passion and bathe in delight
Synchronise your breath with your child each night.
Watch as your baby masters the crawl
Touch the deep sounds of nature's call.
Undefined love, wrapped up in a kiss
Moments so precious no mother could miss.
Challenge the horizons and treasure the view
Free all desires that penetrate you.
Spoil yourself in intuition
Run through obstacles and enjoy the mission.
Search for the meaning in your child's eyes
The truth will shine, as will the lies.
Learn from your child, practise friendship and care
Comfort emotion, speak up and share.
Through good times and bad
Be they happy or sad
Rich or poor
Less or more
Answer the questions deep in your heart
Treat each day as a brand new start.
Hug the presence with all your might
Then close your eyes and sleep tonight.

NATALIE SIMON

Becoming a great parent

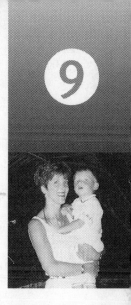

The role of a great parent is to foster their child's self-esteem and a belief that anything is possible.

AS A NEW PARENT, I certainly didn't have the faintest idea where to begin or what to expect. I was an educated woman making my mark on the world, but parenting was a skill I had to learn the hard way, through trial and error. In this chapter I will share with you what I have learnt about being a great parent and the responses to Callum's condition that have been successful.

Being a parent is one of the most important roles that we ever undertake. As parents we provide the blueprint for our children to learn to lead happy and fulfilling lives. It is logical, then, that as parents we need to strive to be the very best we can be. Yet who trains us to fulfil this essential and loving role?

In 2000 a national poll conducted in the United Kingdom by the child helpline association ChildLine (set up by Esther Rantzen) asked, 'Have your parents been good role models?' Only 5 per cent of respondents answered, 'Yes, definitely'. Another question posed by the survey was, 'Would you like to turn out to be like your parents?' Seventy-one per cent of people polled responded with, 'No way'.

Other discouraging statistics reveal that:

- More than 50 000 children in Australia were affected by the divorce of their parents in 1997 and 'almost 1 million children (21 per cent of all children) had one natural parent living outside their household, usually as a consequence of marriage or relationship breakdown' (Australian Bureau of Statistics).[4]
- Of mothers giving birth in Australia in 2000, nearly 5 per cent of them were still teenagers (Australian Bureau of Statistics).[5]
- Research published by the Australian Institute of Criminology demonstrates a direct link between mistreatment of children and juvenile offending. A major study in Queensland in 2003 identified that 23 per cent of children who were victims of physical abuse subsequently offended.[6]
- The 1997 US Census found that 3.9 million children were living in households where a grandparent was the primary caregiver. The most common reasons why children were living with their grandparents were parent drug and alcohol abuse, neglect or abandonment of children, incarceration, physical or mental illness,

death of one or both parents, teenage pregnancy,
divorce or parental unemployment.[7]

These statistics reveal that an alarming number of
parents have difficulty coping with the responsibilities
of parenting a child. It seems to me that we need to break
this cycle.

Western societies have undergone enormous changes.
Women now have the opportunity to enter the workforce
and fulfil the role of 'provider'. Rearing healthy offspring
isn't necessarily our main focus for achieving happiness.
We now have more complex needs for fulfilment: we
strive for pleasure, security, health, variety, love, wealth
and happiness.

Also, the family unit has become smaller, and there are
many different configurations of a 'family'. In the western
world, it's not unusual for a family to have just one child.
According to United Nations figures, 'the world average
total fertility rate for 1995 – 2000 stands at 2.7 babies per
woman'.[8] The *Australian Bureau of Statistics Year Book
2002* states that Australia's total fertility rate for 1999 was
just 1.75 babies per woman, making it 'one of the lowest
in the world'.[9] In instances where the family unit breaks
down, often one partner becomes the sole carer for the
child or children. The pressures on parents today are
unique, and there are many people who are undertaking
this crucial role alone.

So what are the essential steps to being a great parent,
regardless of family background, circumstances or financial
situation? Before you even begin parenting your children,
you need to know:

- how to love yourself
- how to cease feeling guilty
- how to forgive your parents, teachers and friends who put limits on you, and
- how to continually seek to improve yourself.

Building your self-esteem

The most important parenting skill that I have learned is the ability to love unconditionally, and this begins with loving yourself. The healthier your own self-esteem is, the more love and affection you will be able to bestow on your children and other family members. Liking and loving yourself means accepting that you are not perfect and that you will make mistakes.

> Our potential for experiencing happiness and contentment is closely linked to our self-esteem.

It is true that our self-esteem is influenced by our childhood experiences, but the good news is that we can turn negative childhood experiences around and build a healthy self-esteem. Many people manage to lead happy lives in spite of their experiences of inappropriate parenting and other negative external influences. Remember that your past does not equal your future.

Sometimes we reserve our harshest criticism for ourselves. This is a learned response, but it's a habit we can break. Try to remember that you are a special person who deserves to be treasured like a beautiful and rare orchid. Begin by saying to yourself every morning, 'I am beautiful inside and out and I like myself very much.' Make a list of all the things you like doing and do well, and stick your list on the fridge to remind yourself of your qualities whenever you have a low moment. Why not start right now by making a list of all your good points? Consider the following:

- I am a loving parent.
- I am kind and considerate.
- I am a good organiser.
- I am fun to be with.
- I am an industrious worker, artistic and passionate.
- I am a good friend, loyal and beautiful inside and out.

Read your list aloud to yourself every day. Positive action is such a morale booster!

When you really love yourself, you won't set yourself conditions, such as 'I'll love myself *when* I've reached that target at work', or 'I'll love myself *when* I have the perfect look'. These conditions are limiting. Never limit yourself or your children. When you really like yourself, you realise that you can be happy, no matter what your circumstances.

Make an effort with your appearance, even if you feel tired. If you look good, you'll feel good.

Spoil yourself, like yourself and never allow anyone to say anything bad about you. Then as a parent you will foster the same response in your child.

Take regular time out to meditate or simply have a quiet break from your daily tasks. Time out boosts your energy levels, enabling you to be more loving to others. When you are tired, rest. Don't feel you have to keep on going.

Your health and wellbeing should be your first consideration because without them you won't be able to achieve much else. You'll find that you'll feel much happier with life if you rest and take time to 'smell the roses'.

Avoid becoming a martyr. This is a trap that ensnares many parents, especially those of children with special needs. Put yourself first and then you'll have the strength to give to others. This is not vanity or selfishness; it is essential for you to be able to continue loving and giving consistently.

Once you really start to follow these pieces of advice, you'll feel like a heavy weight has been lifted from your shoulders.

Discarding feelings of guilt

If you think about it, guilt is simply negative, wasted energy. It really is a waste of your time and precious energy to feel guilty about anything. The past is behind you and it has no relevance to or bearing on the present or the future, except as a lesson. Say to yourself:

As of this moment, I have a clean slate.
I cannot undo what has been done;
I can only learn a lesson and move on.

Many people with low self-esteem tend to throw guilt at others, criticise or complain, and load their problems onto people they consider friends. This increases the weight of their own burdens, as they end up carrying other people's problems as well as their own.

If you are doing anything in your life because of guilt, stop and look at the situation. Ask yourself whether doing this thing, whatever it is, will lift your spirits and be of benefit to anyone, including yourself. Will it have a detrimental effect by disempowering you? I'm not suggesting that you avoid doing anything you don't like doing, but do take responsibility for your actions and endeavour to do everything with passion and enthusiasm.

> The best way to do anything is by doing it because *you really want to.*

Loving your child unconditionally

The most important parenting skill that I have learnt is the ability to love unconditionally. Loving our children unconditionally means loving them no matter whether they are healthy or disabled, well-behaved or naughty, happy or irritable, achieve low or high grades at school, choose friends we approve of or disapprove of, or whether they fulfil our dreams for them or disappoint us in some way. Loving unconditionally means never threatening to withdraw our love from our children.

When I asked Rory and a group of his friends 'what does love mean?' they gave the following answers:

Mummys and daddys in love get married.
                              Didi Lambert, aged five

People show they love you with hugs and kisses. I'm in love with Angie, my sister.
                              Krystopher Glindemann, aged five

Mums and dads show they love you by buying you food and nice things for your bedroom.
                              Audrey Hanna, aged six

People who love you kiss and hug you. Mums and dads in love sleep together.
                              Mathew Lambert, aged seven

You know people are in love when they kiss like '007'.
                              Jonathon Glindemann, aged eight

Love is a very special thing. If someone was to love you, they would have to make you feel warm and special, give you hugs and kisses and not leave you out.
                              Chardonnay Hanna, aged nine

Love is opposite to hatred. I love my mum to the sun, moon, stars, England, Spain, Australia and back again, 589 trillion million times!
                              Rory Sykes, aged ten

Love is caring for each other.
Angela Glindemann, aged 11

To love someone, you must appreciate being
with them, spend time together, and care and
be there for them in times of need.
Chavez Hanna, aged 12

My friend Jon recently told me about one of his family members in England who has a young son born left-handed. The boy's father told his son that it is bad manners to use his left hand and insisted that the boy use his right hand at all times. Of course the boy was clumsy with his right hand and lacked coordination. The father repeatedly told his son how clumsy he was and how disappointed he was with the boy's poor handwriting and sporting ability. The boy was sent off to boarding school to be taught some self-control! As a result he developed low self-esteem and became withdrawn and introverted. He believed that he was hopeless at sport, until Jon took this young boy out to play cricket one day and encouraged him to hit and throw the ball with his right hand. It turns out that the boy is a gifted sportsman when permitted to use the right hand that he favours.

Parents need to love their children unconditionally rather than placing limits on them. It is hardly surprising that psychologists tell us it can take 40 years to get over the first five years of our lives.

To some extent parents today have become focused on providing their children with the latest technological gadgets at the expense of simple parenting principles for raising happy children. We can easily fall into the trap of believing that unless we provide our children with the latest in computer technology, the best clothes or the most expensive education, we are not being a good parent. However, providing expensive items and top-of-the-range schooling for our children is no substitute for giving them unconditional love and spending time with them. Providing both is ideal, but being a great parent is achievable no matter what financial resources you have at your disposal. When Rory was only little, I didn't have enough money to spare for birthday presents, so one year I gave him string, Blu-Tac, ribbon and cellophane in a shoe box. Rory was delighted. He set about inventing, tying string between doors and creating a 'web' and cubby holes. He played for hours. Naturally I was caught up in his imaginary games!

Forgiving the negative people in your life

Okay, you say, but how can I love unconditionally when my own parents, teachers or friends have discouraged me or criticised me in some way? The answer is that at some point we have to break this negative cycle by forgiving anyone who has been a negative influence in our lives. We have to move on with life. In order to forgive others we need to be generous in spirit. Remember that the people who criticised you, who were negative or who limited you in some way are human like you, ploughing through life in the best way they can. Give them credit for getting you to this point, whether it is directly or by default.

Seeking to improve yourself

It's important to recognise that happiness comes from within. Throughout my years of personal development and my experiences with Rory, I have learnt that happiness is a personal choice we make, regardless of external conditions.

> If you are unhappy inside, your unhappiness travels with you.

For inspiration, try reading biographies and auto-biographies of people you admire to see how they have achieved their life goals. Many people have triumphed against enormous odds and turned their lives around, becoming happy and fulfilled people. Sometimes we imagine that other people are leading 'perfect' lives, but when you scratch beneath the surface, you often learn that they have experienced their fair share of difficulties and hurdles. Remember that it is not what happens to you in life that counts, but the way you respond to life events.

Reading *Being Happy* by Andrew Matthews really motivated and inspired me. It reassured me that my doubts and fears were normal and okay. It helped me to live through the experiences of raising a disabled boy as a single mum with joy and confidence. I began to realise how lucky I was to have high self-esteem and such confidence. I was able to feel grateful that I had this strength, and also understand the ways in which it could be damaged or whittled away by the cruel or thoughtless comments of others. I realised that I had to protect my special gift and ensure that I helped to raise the self-esteem of those around me.

Continue to develop your interests and abilities by learning from others, reading, taking courses and spending time on your hobbies. Whether you enjoy gardening, playing sport, music, painting, learning a language, taking an evening course, spending time with family and friends, or simply taking a walk, make sure you keep up these enjoyable activities. Our children learn from our example, so we can demonstrate to them how to create a life that is varied and interesting, one that helps us to feel balanced, happy and fulfilled. Remember too that your happiness is contagious.

> I hear and I forget,
> I see and I remember.
> I do and I understand.
> CONFUCIOUS

Building your child's self-esteem

There are a number of ways in which we can help to build our child's self-esteem. The most important of these, of course, is to love them unconditionally, to tell them regularly how much we love them and to continually emphasise how beautiful they are inside and out. Other strategies for improving the self-esteem of a child with a disability or with special needs include:

Giving children empowering 'stories'

One of my strategies for fostering Rory's self-esteem was to give him 'stories' that he could use to explain his condition to others. I thought it was most important to give Rory a story to explain his legs to new friends, mainly to keep his self-esteem high. A story helps a child to realise that the circumstances of their disability aren't their fault. Children tend to blame themselves for anything that is not 'right' or 'normal', from disability to divorce to a parent being cross or tired. A story gives the child permission to like themselves!

I had been teased at school about my different-coloured eyes until Mum told me that they made me special and I was an 'Egyptian princess'. Every girl at school wanted eyes like mine after that! Of course with Rory everyone has always asked what's wrong with his legs. I thought it was important for him to feel 'normal'. Children want to be like all the other children, and I wanted Rory to mix with all kinds of children, not just those with disabilities. I felt that he would benefit from being as much like the children in his social circle as possible. This is the story I created for him to explain to other children about his legs:

> You were in my tummy having a lovely time, all cozy and snuggly. Then your mum was involved in a car accident. Carbooom! You shouted, 'Oh, Mum, what are you doing out there? Oh, my poor head ... oh, my poor legs!'
>
> Poor Mum had injured her tummy and cracked her sternum. She was covered in cuts and bruises.

Being a boy, Rory thought this was an excellent story. I had to repeat it for him many times over. Now he is able to retell the tale perfectly, and so can his friends. Kids are mesmerised by stories like that one. They can all relate to cars and injury. If anyone new asks Rory what's wrong with his legs, the other children answer for him, 'Oh, he was in a car accident.' This gives Rory back his 'normality' and it sounds like an exciting adventure, which makes him a leader of the pack. It means that he seems special to himself and to those he wants to impress. It really works.

I also created a story for another child with cerebral palsy:

> You were in your mummy's tummy, saying, 'Let me out! Let me out!'. Your dad was trying to hurry and get her gently into the car to take you both to the hospital. He raced you to the hospital, and when you finally got there the doctors put your mum on a bed and wheeled her into an operating theatre. You were still yelling, 'Let me out! Let me out! I can't breathe and there is a thick food cord wrapped around my neck!'
>
> It was awful. Eventually the doctors managed to help you out of your mummy's tummy, so you could breathe, but you had already missed out on a lot of air. You were so lucky to be alive, and your parents were so lucky that you hadn't died in your mummy's tummy. You were born a lucky person. Despite the cerebral palsy, you are safe and well.

Rory's stories helped to empower him in difficult situations and to not think of himself as 'disabled'. Once people Rory met were given an explanation for his condition, they would generally accept him for who he was and not think of him as someone with a disability.

Demonstrating positive reactions

Children don't often have preconceived ideas about how they must behave, react or respond to different situations. They simply react instinctively until they are taught how to react by parents, teachers or older siblings.

For instance, in a group of preschool-aged children playing together, some children might be white, some black, and some may have a disability like Rory's. The physical characteristics of the other children don't really matter to their playmates; they simply play together and accept things as they are. Of course they are curious and will ask questions like: 'Why are you white when I am black?' or 'Why do you walk funny?' But if a child gives them an explanation, usually the subject is closed and they move on. The biases and prejudices we experience as adults are a learned response.

Prejudice often arises from fear and ignorance. Time and time again over the years, many people had ignored Rory and me. They truly didn't know how to respond to our differences. Some people would talk to me as if Rory wasn't there and ask me what was wrong with him, as if he couldn't hear them. I would respond by saying, 'Rory is a miracle surviving a car crash. Look how well he is walking with his calipers ... Show them, Rory.' On cue, Rory would strut his stuff in his wobbly fashion, or do a wheelie in his wheelchair, depending on what stage he had reached. The person looking on would be open-mouthed and usually shocked at the answer, but would always agree with me when I said, 'He's doing well, isn't he?' This response boosted Rory's self-esteem.

Helping your child to reach their potential

Depending on the level of learning challenges or disability that your child experiences, it may well be possible to integrate them into a 'regular' school environment so that they can socialise with children both with and without disabilities. Investigate the schooling options that are available to your child, and visit the various schools to ascertain which one will best assist your child to reach their potential. Even if your child is unable to attend a 'regular' school, try to provide them with opportunities to make friends and mix with children both with and without special needs.

Encourage your child to participate in activities that they enjoy and which give them confidence and boost

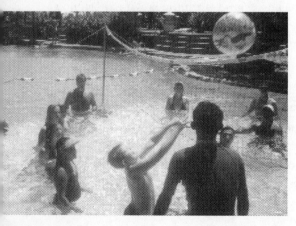

'I'll get it!'

their self-esteem. Don't limit them just because they have hurdles to overcome to achieve their goals. Rory has always loved swimming, dancing, horse-riding, practising his golf on the driving range, and participating in school sports. He would join in with me when I was relaxing by painting, drawing or learning about feng shui. He became a whiz on the computer, enjoys playing computer games and has always attended his friends' parties. We encourage his friends to come over to our place, take them with us on outings and have sleep-overs. Rory has been able to experience all the activities that children without cerebral palsy enjoy.

Assisting your child to look their best

We all seem to be attracted to beautiful things and beautiful people. Young children always seem to prefer the teacher with blonde hair, long legs, big eyes and pretty clothes compared to the less glamorous teacher who is such a kind person. Unfortunately it is a fact that western societies are fixated with youth and beauty. I believe that it is essential to ensure that our children look the best they possibly can to fit in with society's image of what is 'normal'.

Because cosmetic surgery has become commonplace among the rich and famous, many people now regard it as nothing more than an act of vanity. However, this disregards the very worthwhile applications of cosmetic or plastic surgery in assisting children and adults to achieve the best appearance for them, one that is regarded as 'normal' in the eyes of society. It can be such a boost to a child's self-esteem for them to undergo surgery to fix cosmetic problems. In many cases the benefits are not only physical and medical, but also psychological. A child's age and type of disability determine the surgical options that may be available to them. I believe that responsible use of cosmetic or plastic surgery can help prevent unnecessary suffering. Remember that mental suffering can be just as painful as physical suffering.

Rory now has good vision, no glasses and no sign of a squint unless he is tired. His surgery was performed when he was a baby, so he has no memories of the trauma. I felt it more keenly than he did – I felt sick to the stomach for days before his eye surgery. But I have no regrets. It was certainly worth it.

If possible, arrange for your child to have surgery while still an infant so that they are spared the teasing that occurs at school, and that can have a detrimental effect on a small child's psyche. Don't let your child suffer any more than is unavoidable.

Children want to be just like everyone else. They don't appreciate being different. Anyone who was overweight as a child will know what it is like to be 'different' and picked on. Children with large, sticking-out ears are picked on, and yet it is such a simple operation to correct. If your child has a large birthmark on their face, ask a surgeon what can be done. If there is no surgery that can help, tell your child how beautiful they are and that they have a special, magical mark like Harry Potter! Give them a reason to be proud of what marks them out as different – just like I felt when my mother told me I was an Egyptian princess because of my different coloured eyes. In 2000, a Maltese couple became parents to conjoined ('Siamese') twin girls. At first the mother found it hard to even look at the girls as they were so unlike the children of her dreams. She cried a lot, and felt bad about herself, but gradually, the more she touched and held each little girl's hand, the more she realised that each girl had her own personality. Only then did the mother begin to bond with her girls.

In this very rare case, the family's tragic story was made into a TV documentary. The twins were operated on to separate them, but in order for either of the girls to survive, one would have to die. The strongest twin, despite looking quite abnormal at birth, underwent cosmetic and corrective surgery. She was transformed into the child that the couple had originally hoped for. After a rough start to life, she now has the chance of leading a happy, healthy life with her devoted parents, an outcome that may have seemed impossible when she was born. This example is amazing because it takes disfigurement at its most unusual and yet shows you that anything is possible, and it is normal to have conflicting emotions.

To this day, I feel extremely blessed that my life plan brought me into the health and wellbeing industry. I instinctively felt that I had a purpose in life and something to offer others. I knew I could make a difference by helping others to feel good about themselves. After spending each day beautifying healthy, gorgeous people, it became apparent to me that many people develop poor self-esteem. A significant part of my role at my health spas was to counsel and boost the morale of my clients. It is obvious to me that if healthy and able-bodied people feel bad about themselves then how much greater are the hurdles that have to be overcome by people with obvious physical disabilities?

Giving your child 'living lessons'

It had always been my dream that if I ever became a mother I would be in a position to take my children around the world in order to teach them about history, geography and sociology by experiencing different cultures first hand.

I decided that Rory wouldn't miss out on any of the fun activities that he would have experienced if he had been born without cerebral palsy and if my marriage had remained intact. By the time he was six months old Rory had travelled to Jamaica and visited friends in Switzerland. At the age of one he travelled around the world to Singapore, New Zealand and Australia.

You may not have the means to travel or enjoy the sorts of holidays that Rory and I have been lucky to experience together. But no matter what your financial circumstances are, you can make life enjoyable by

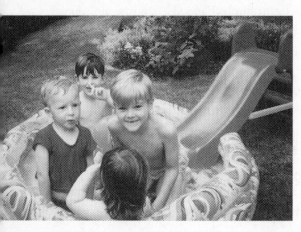

Not quite a pool, but very sociable!

creating a loving atmosphere at home, taking regular inexpensive outings in your local area and making your child's daily routine and exercise program as varied and fun as possible. Despite our low finances after my divorce we would still invite all our friends over to celebrate our joint birthday. Use whatever means you have at your disposal to make your life interesting and enjoyable.

Creating a loving atmosphere at home

> A loving atmosphere at home
> is the foundation for your life.
> DALAI LAMA

To keep both Rory's and my spirits up, I aim to always create a loving home environment – a home that has an atmosphere of warmth and is welcoming to others. I regularly invite both Rory's and my friends over, which fills our home with laughter and energy. Entertaining at home needn't be expensive. It can be as simple as inviting someone over for a drink and a chat, a barbecue in the backyard, or to watch TV. I make a habit of doing activities at home that I enjoy, and encourage Rory to do the same. For relaxation I love to read and paint.

Whenever I am feeling low, I find the following strategies helpful:

- Block out any negativity. Stay away from friends and family who bring you down and surround yourself with the positive people in your life.

- Watch happy films and TV programs rather than focusing on disturbing news and world events.
- Surround yourself with pleasant smells and sights. Turn the radio or stereo to upbeat music, or music that makes you feel relaxed.
- Go for a walk in the park, by a river, lake, or by the sea.

These things are possible no matter what your financial situation. For me, laughter is the best cure for any ailment, from exhaustion to feeling low. I think it's what gives me my high energy levels and the zest to cram as many exciting things into my daily life as possible.

Home should feel like the haven we can return to after our busy day at work or at school, a place where we can put aside the demands of the world and recharge our batteries. It should be a true reflection of our bright personalities.

Discipline and the difficult child

Let's face it, raising a child is frequently very demanding and challenging, especially when it comes to providing appropriate parameters and discipline. Finding the balance between discipline and love can be very challenging. Dealing with the frustrations and tantrums of a child, and especially one with special needs, brings its own challenges. But it is important to remember that a child with special needs should be treated in the same way that you would treat any other child, with love, acceptance and clear guidelines.

Many children, particularly those with a disability, may experience quite intense feelings of anger and frustration at being unable to do the things that other children do. They may take their frustration out on themselves by hurting themselves, which is awful to witness. Rory would sometimes thump his legs or bang his head on the wall. I would admonish him with strong words, hugging him tightly at the same time and saying, 'How dare you hurt yourself when Mummy has taken so much time and effort to make you strong and well? When you hurt yourself you are hurting your mum and you don't want to hurt Mummy.' Mind you, if they do want to hurt you, they may continue. Always ask what it is that has made them cross.

It can be difficult to develop a child's confidence if they need help with simple tasks or if many things must be done for them. Rory would say to me, 'I'm no good. I can't walk.' I wanted to cry, but instead I would take Rory and 'make' him walk around the house with me, holding him up and saying: 'There you go, you *can* walk around the house. You've just done it.' Even though it wasn't what he really meant, he would laugh because he knew I was trying to get him there and he *had* just walked around the house, in a manner of speaking.

It's essential to help your child to do as much as possible for themselves and to feel a sense of achievement for all the successes they have, no matter how small. Give them lots of positive feedback and praise to help them feel good about themselves and to encourage them to keep striving to achieve new goals.

I have always told Rory what lovely long legs he has, and that he has the most beautiful hair colouring and beautiful skin. I tell him regularly that he is so handsome, I want to kiss him!

Just like any other child, a child with a disability will exhibit behavioural problems from time to time. Appropriate discipline and setting limits for your children are just as important in nurturing their self-esteem as unconditional love and acceptance. Setting clear boundaries and rules for our children helps them to feel protected. Discipline is essential for our children to learn about socially acceptable behaviour that will assist them to get along with other people.

After Rory's seventh birthday party, my parenting skills were really put to the test. He had had a wonderful time with his friends, but he was tired. He worked himself into a tantrum outside the house because I wouldn't allow him to do something. He was making such a horrendous screaming noise that people were stopping in the street to see if he was being attacked. I tried my usual tactic of counting to ten. This generally worked, because Rory knew that when I reached 'ten' I would really get cross. This time it didn't work. I have no excuse other than being a tired single mum who had just done her best for her son's birthday party … I smacked him. Immediately I felt terrible. Rory was shocked too. After profuse apologies to Rory for losing control, I sat down with him and explained that parents aren't perfect and they're not always right. Parents have rules that they believe will make things safe and enjoyable for the family, and each member of the family has to take responsibility for playing their part. Rory said it was still wrong of me to have smacked him. True. So when I asked him what he thought I should have done when he ignored my count to ten, he said, 'Simple. Count to 20.'

Children make you lose your patience sometimes, but they also make you laugh. They're smart too, and rationalising with them really works.

I explained to Rory that arranging parties and taking him on outings and holidays really put a strain on me, but I enjoyed doing it because it made a difference to his life, especially when he laughed a lot and had fun. He understood, and we hugged and made up.

It is vital to discipline children in a positive manner. Negative discipline is likely to only make things worse. Don't give in to a child's temper tantrums. Tell them that the behaviour is unacceptable and must stop. If necessary, tell them that they will not be allowed to watch a favourite TV program or that some other treat will be denied. Under no circumstances should you threaten to withdraw your love for them, but you must follow through with your threat to deny them a treat if they continue to behave badly. They soon catch on.

There are other behavioural difficulties that may be associated with a child with special needs. If they have difficulty communicating with others they may demand a lot of attention from their parents. It is possible to maintain contact with your child while you are doing other things, simply by talking to them frequently and making eye contact. When Rory was a baby and couldn't see, I would carry him around with me in a papoose so that he would feel comforted by my presence. I also would play calming music and surround us with pleasant scents so that his other senses were engaged. It made life more interesting for him and prevented boredom and anxiety.

Boredom can be a significant problem for children, especially those with a disability (particularly if their mobility is limited) or children with high intelligence. Try to involve them in as many activities as possible, and encourage other children to come to your house to play. Always encourage your child to be a fully active participant in life, to adopt socially acceptable behaviours, to make decisions and choices and to think for themself, just as you would any other child. Remember that your goal is to give your child as close to a normal life as possible.

Siblings

Siblings of a child with special needs or of a new baby may feel jealous of the attention that the baby or disabled child receives from the parents. They may also feel embarrassed or ashamed of their sibling. It is important to

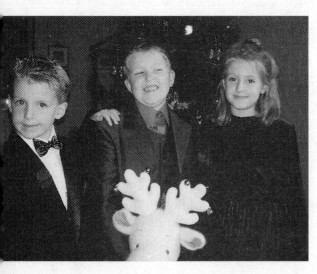

Callum with his cousins, Sebastian and Amber. Beverley Hills kids, eat your heart out!

explain the child's condition to their siblings and help them to learn to accept any differences. This is another area where giving children 'stories' to explain why their brother or sister has special needs can really help.

It is equally important to treat all the children in the family in the same loving way and to include them all in outings, treats and holidays. Children are remarkably adept at discerning any differences in treatment that they may receive. Don't assume that because a child is very young they don't notice if they are being ignored or treated differently to their brothers or sisters.

A great parent differentiates between their children to suit each child's personality.

Siblings can be an enormous help in assisting a child with special needs to develop new skills and try things

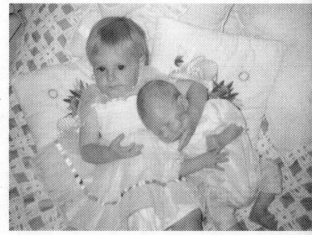

Amber taking care of Callum. 'Mum, she's got me in a headlock!'

for themselves. Just as younger children copy their older siblings, a child with special needs can learn a lot from their siblings.

Encourage them to be as independent as possible so that their siblings do not regard them as a burden.

Siblings of a child with special needs can really benefit, as they often develop a maturity and sense of responsibility that other children of their age simply don't possess. They can also acquire an understanding of and appreciation for good health that other children might not develop for many years.

Remember that if you are experiencing difficulties in coping with any aspects of your child's behaviour or development, seek help rather than suffering in silence or allowing yourself to reach desperation point. There are many organisations that can help you deal with your particular circumstances (see page 227–232). The chances are that many other people are in similar circumstances to you and you can benefit from their experiences and learn approaches that have worked for them. You are never alone.

Adolescents: learning to let go

Our children are not possessions for us to hold onto, or an investment for ourselves in later years. As children reach adolescence it is quite normal for them to switch off from the influence of their parents and begin to form their own judgments and make their own decisions. This is an essential step to becoming an adult.

As children reach adolescence and push for more independence, it is still important for parents to set a great example for them. If you don't want your kids to smoke, abuse alcohol or drugs, then let them see you leading a healthy life. Lead by example.

Many teenagers say that they don't feel heard or understood. A great parent will listen and acknowledge that their teenager has a different viewpoint and one that is not necessarily wrong.

> A great parent shows respect for their teenager's thoughts and ideas, even if they don't agree with them.

Give emotional support to your teenager: be proud of them when they make wise decisions, and comfort them when the consequences of their decisions are not quite what they expected.

If at any time your values are compromised by your teenager's actions, then your teenager should be made aware of this through rational communication. Convey to them that while they are under your care they need to respect your values, in the same way that a guest is expected to respect the wishes of their host while they are under their roof.

> A great parent tries to keep up with their teenager's passions and interests.

Give your teenager the encouragement to experiment with new styles and fashions, to make new friends and try new sports and other activities. If your child already has a solid foundation of high self-esteem, confidence and the knowledge that they are loved unconditionally, they will have begun to develop high standards for themselves.

I am a firm believer that all adolescents should be taught how to be great parents too, while they are still at school, so that they gain some insight into the responsibilities of parenting and may develop a less defiant attitude towards their parents.

A great parent learns to let go of their teenager and encourages independence. This is never easy to do, but if we give our children the freedom to fly, then they will willingly return to the nest for a visit. I still have a few years to go before Rory will be leaving me, but I know it will be an adjustment for me. However, witnessing his excitement at experiencing new adventures will be comforting. He has already told me he will sing 'Mama, I never want to hurt you' by Eminem when he leaves home. I responded that I would not be hurt because it was healthy to leave home and that I would even help design his new place if he wanted. Of course I would expect him to invite me over to his place for one of his delicious meals ... He is a great cook!

Drawing up an action plan

We are what we repeatedly do.
Excellence then is not an act, but a habit.
ARISTOTLE

Mind you, stupidity is doing the same thing, over and over, yet expecting a different result!

You will never accomplish more than you set out to accomplish. We need to put ourselves in a position to influence the things that happen in our lives. Excuses, distractions and fear are all part of life. If we acknowledge that they exist and are a normal part of being human, we can plan to remove each obstacle from our path, systematically, one by one.

- Plan to be what you know you can be: to be easy to live with, loving, kind and fun.
- Plan to do what you know you can do: serve others and bring joy to those you love.
- Plan to have what you know you can have: wealth, happiness, love, security, health, pleasure and success.

It is such a relief when you finally make a decision to do something. Action removes any fears.

On many occasions since Rory was a baby, I have simply had to make a conscious decision to act, in order to preserve my sanity. For instance, I made the decision to persist with Rory's eye patching and do whatever else it would take to give him every chance of being able to see. I decided to believe that it was possible. My belief became my reality.

I was told that babies do not see much for the first six weeks. After about six weeks they begin to have more focus, and their eyes then continue to develop over the next seven years. So I knew that we had until Rory was seven to give him the very best chance of achieving good vision. I was unwilling to waste one minute. Every day for seven years Rory had his eyes patched to help the eye muscles to strengthen and develop. Many mums I met during that time stopped patching their child's eyes after only a few weeks, or were not consistent with the patching. It was part of Rory's routine and we made it into a game. Rory took action by deciding to play along with this game.

Children sense very early on if they are different in some way from other children. My confidence and faith was infectious. Rory knew that he was going to see and run.

Whatever we strive towards, we can achieve.

Remain open to opportunities that arise, and create your own opportunities. You never know who is around the corner to inspire you or to take you to the next stage of personal development. It is important, however, to always keep in mind your child's dreams and desires. They might not be the same as your own, and their dreams are more important than your desires where their life is concerned. If you can dream it, you can achieve it.

Dream and plant the seed in your child's mind
that everything is possible.

Setting goals and objectives

A goal is a dream in action, with a purpose. Goals should be specific, solid and serious. They need to have deadlines, otherwise they are just dreams rather than plans in motion. Success at achieving goals doesn't require a super intellect. Success is making the best of who we are.

I once saw an old man being interviewed on TV on his 102nd birthday. The reporter asked him if he had any regrets. The man responded by saying that he wished he had looked after his body while he was younger; if he had known he was going to live so long, he would have taken better care of himself! He also regretted not having taken more chances in life rather than doing what he believed was expected of him. The reporter then asked whether he had any advice to offer younger people. The old man said, 'Look after your health and enjoy the present day. Don't worry about the future, but live each day to the full as if it were your last. Then you'll have no regrets.'

This is wise advice, indeed, for us all to heed. Don't worry what other people think. Do what you know is right for you and your family. Follow your own path.

Often we forget to focus on our dreams and fall into a routine of just living day after day without excitement and energy. We lose our sparkle. This is why goals and objectives are so important. They keep us focused. We have something worthwhile to aim for, and we can enjoy the day knowing that we are heading towards something positive.

Throughout Rory's therapy program we would sit down together every week and determine his weekly and monthly objectives. It is important to set realistic timeframes for children to achieve their goals. Achievement of goals builds a child's self-esteem and confidence.

If you were asked what you would do if you won the lottery, what would be your response? Write down a list of activities you would do, places you would visit, and charities you would support.

My list would include donating 10 per cent to family, friends and charity, buying a pale-yellow 911 cabriolet Porsche, a waterfront house, going on a world cruise, investing some money, continuing to write and work on TV programs, and employing a cook and a tutor for Rory.

Now, if you were told that you only had six months to live (in which time you would remain healthy and then suddenly pop your clogs), what would you do in those six months? Write down what your response would be.

When I did this exercise some years ago, I wrote down that I would sell up our home and my business in England and travel around the world with Rory, visiting friends and making new ones.

All the activities you wrote down in answer to these questions should also appear on your list of goals and objectives. Don't wait for retirement, a lottery win or having just a few months to live before focusing on what you really want to achieve in life.

Anything is possible!

Children need to experience the feeling that anything is possible and that whatever goal they set their mind to they can achieve. Encourage realistic goal setting and praise them for all the milestones they reach, no matter how small or insignificant they may seem. Do not limit their goals, but encourage positive thinking and independence.

I truly believe that Callum has helped me to become a more passionate and caring person, which in turn has increased my happiness enormously. Callum, on the other hand, has been lucky to have me as his mother, to encourage him, love him unconditionally and always believe in him.

ABCs of Life's Journey

As an exceptional traveller on the road of life you will:

Appreciate who you are

Be nice to everybody

Choose your own road

Dodge negativity

Envision your destination

Flaunt your fabulousness

Go where your heart leads

Have faith

Investigate life's twists and turns

Jump!

Keep on keeping on

Love lots

Make friends

Never litter

Observe the scenery

Play often

Quit worrying

Relax

Stop and smell the flowers

Take it one step at a time

Unload your excess baggage

Venture into the unknown

Walk a mile in someone else's shoes

X-pect the best

Yield to fun

Zone out occasionally, it's good for you

Anonymous

Devising a program for your child

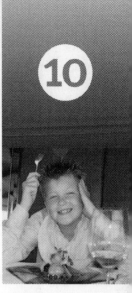

To lose one's health renders
science null, art inglorious,
strength unavailing, wealth
useless and eloquence powerless.

Hemophilus

RORY HAS OVERCOME some tremendous
physical problems through consistent and disciplined
effort. Rory's experiences show that anything is possible
if you have a goal and strive for it. Don't let other people
limit you, even if their remarks are motivated by goodwill.
Surround yourself with positive, successful people so that
you can learn from their experiences.

Our attitude and the way we respond to life events is a significant contributing factor to our sense of happiness and wellbeing. Just as important as encouraging a healthy, positive attitude to life is the way in which diet and exercise influence our health and happiness. In conjunction with the use of therapy supervised by various medical professionals, this chapter discusses the benefits of diet, exercise and medical therapies in your child's development.

Conventional medical therapies

The contribution of a team of health professionals is invaluable in developing an appropriate program to assist your child's development. In Rory's case, we relied very much on the efforts of physiotherapists, orthoptists, ophthalmologists, psychologists and numerous doctors

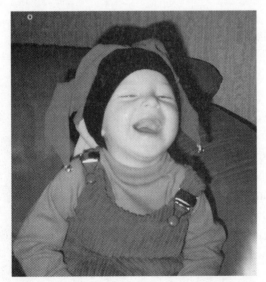

Laughter is the best medicine

and surgeons. Encouraging your child to reach their full potential is a team effort.

A child with cerebral palsy may experience multiple disabilities, including vision problems, hearing difficulties, speech and language problems and learning disabilities. It is important that your child is fully assessed by a team of medical specialists to ascertain what therapy will best assist them.

Early intervention is essential if your child is to have the best chance of leading a normal life. Physical therapy should begin as soon as a child is diagnosed with cerebral palsy. Your family doctor or paediatrician will refer you to the appropriate therapy services.

Remember that therapists cannot 'cure' cerebral palsy, but they can certainly help to reduce the effects of the condition. People with cerebral palsy are affected in different ways and to varying degrees. Everyone can

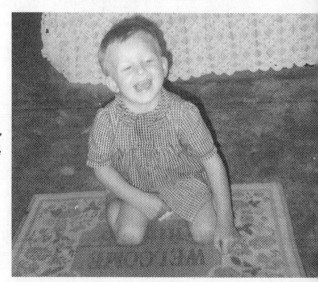

'Now I can sit up!'
Callum aged 2½

achieve improvements, but not every child with cerebral palsy will achieve the same outcomes.

Physical therapy aims to achieve three important outcomes: preventing muscles from becoming rigid and fixed in awkward positions, preventing the weakening and deterioration of muscles through lack of use, and improving the child's motor skills. Therapists will work closely with you and/or your child's carers to demonstrate how you can help your child with daily activities and with play that will boost their development. They will advise you at each stage of development which types of toys will encourage learning, and show you the most effective ways of handling your child. The team of therapists will plan ahead and set realistic goals to ensure that your child

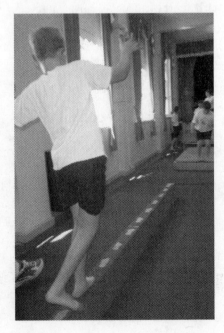

'Look at me now! Olympics 2004, here I come!'

develops the essential movements necessary for each stage of development and is helped to participate in life as fully as possible.

A child with cerebral palsy will experience delayed development because the brain, which controls all movements, has been damaged. Unlike an able-bodied child, who will move quite easily and naturally from one stage of development to the next, a child with cerebral palsy may miss some of the stages of development. For instance, if the child is unable to lie on their tummy, they may not learn the steps to sit up by first using their neck muscles to lift their head, supporting themselves with their arms, and then using their back and neck muscles to push themselves up. Without developing these abilities they won't naturally progress to being able to stand up.

Similarly, if they experience limited movement in the lower limbs, they may have to use their arms instead of their legs to push themselves along the ground, which could result in stiffening and bending of the arms, making it difficult for them to learn to stretch and reach out for things.

Whatever program of exercises and therapy is recommended by your child's team of therapists, persisting with the program and repeating the exercises regularly will greatly improve your child's progress. It is likely that much of the work with your child will need to be done at home. Try to think of the team of therapists as 'coaches' who guide you through the necessary program and push your child to reach their potential. Like an athlete, your child needs to practise and train every day in order to improve, and they need your constant encouragement.

Some of the parents of children with cerebral palsy undergoing therapy at the same time as Rory became disillusioned when they didn't see early results, and therefore didn't persist with the daily home exercise program because they felt it wasn't beneficial. However, I am convinced that the regular repetitive program of exercises that we undertook at home played a significant role in helping Rory to learn to walk and run. If progress is slow, therapists will help to ease any frustration that you or your child experience and to reassure you that this is normal. Don't give up if early signs are discouraging. Your child's determination and family support are two very important factors determining whether they will achieve their long-term goals.

If at any time you are unhappy with an assessment or treatment that your child receives, seek another opinion or contact one of the support organisations listed on pages 227–230 for assistance.

Physiotherapy

A physiotherapist will evaluate and treat mobility difficulties associated with problems in the muscles and bones. They use methods such as exercise, manipulation, heat and ultrasonic treatments, and massage. They will show you how to lift and carry your child properly and position them in the best way to promote good movement and muscle development.

Cerebral palsy often causes muscles to tighten, becoming stiff and rigid. This 'spasticity' is caused by damage to the motor area of the brain. If this part of the cerebral cortex is damaged, it affects the way in which nerve signals travel along the spinal cord through the nervous system to the tendons and muscles, including muscles in the arms, legs, fingers and toes, as well as the eye and mouth muscles. Spasticity can be a very painful condition.

The physiotherapist will teach your child ways of minimising muscle stiffness and demonstrate effective movements by using a program of exercises. They may also introduce the use of splints. They will demonstrate an exercise program for you to do regularly with your child at home. They will assess and demonstrate the best sitting and walking patterns, and may help to improve your child's posture. Pictured above is the personal exercise program developed for Rory when he was seven.

As described in Chapter 5, I did my very best at all times to ensure that Rory's physiotherapy exercises were enjoyable. This wasn't always easy, as by their very

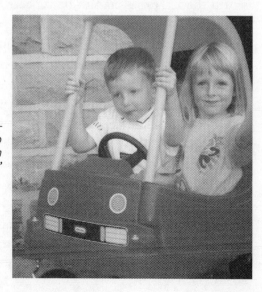

'Amber's the engine –
my feet won't go
where I want them
to yet.'

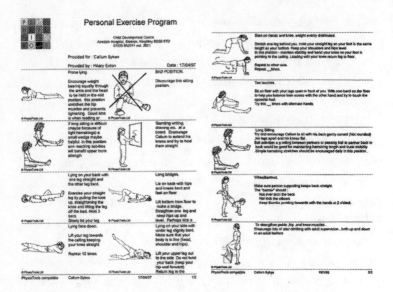

'That doesn't look like me at all, Mum!' Callum's physiotherapy cards

nature the exercises had to be repeated many times to be effective, and some of the constant pushing down on Rory's leg muscles could be quite painful for him. Rory's physiotherapist, Ruth McAlister, was very supportive of my adaptations to her exercise program, encouraging me when I decided to try putting his tight little thighs around my hips and dancing around with him to stretch his leg muscles. This is where imagination really counts. Each person can develop an exciting program to suit his or her life and environment. Don't ever feel constrained by the advice of doctors or of 'do-gooders'. There are no limits to your imagination. And remember, you don't have to do it all on your own. When your child's friends come for sleep-overs or to play, they can assist you with massaging your child and create their own games. It all helps.

It took two and a half years for Rory to learn how to crawl. It really does take a lot of time and effort for a child with cerebral palsy to master a new pattern of movement, but once it is imprinted in the mind, it stays. Rory's small progressions gave me the faith and enthusiasm to persist with his daily exercise program. A weekly physiotherapy session is not sufficient to overcome spasticity, so do not rely solely on the sessions supervised by your child's physiotherapist. The more effort and energy you put into your child's daily physiotherapy, the greater the results will be. Never give up, no matter how tired you are. Ask for help from friends and family. You may be surprised how other people, especially children, like to help out.

Occupational therapy

An occupational therapist will assess and treat physical problems and assist your child to function effectively at home and in the wider community. They can provide suitable equipment for your child and recommend adaptations to your home and your child's school environment to facilitate daily activities and your child's independence. They can also advise on suitable play equipment and other aids, such as trolleys to assist mobility.

One of the most important adaptations we had made at home was a special wooden box with handles that fitted around the toilet once Rory became too big for a potty. This enabled him to gain stability to accomplish this significant task on his own, and it boosted his self-esteem because it made him feel like a big boy.

The other major change that really helped Rory once he was able to begin walking with some assistance was the fitting of a handrail to the side of the house and to our steep drive This gave him some independence and saved me from having to carry him into the house as he grew and became heavier.

Speech and language therapy

If your child experiences difficulties in using or understanding spoken and written language, they will be referred to a speech and language therapist, who will help them to maximise communication skills. These therapists may be involved at a very early stage if your child exhibits problems feeding, drinking or swallowing, skills that are important not only for the child's health and nutrition, but ultimately for learning to produce speech sounds.

Tightened mouth muscles can cause problems with speech and make the sufferer drool, which may lead others to falsely assume that they are intellectually disabled. A child with cerebral palsy may have delayed speech because they don't have the same ability to play and explore that other children have. If your child has significant difficulties with speech and language development, they may be assisted with a communication device that augments or replaces speech, such as a communication board.

On page 83 I describe how I taught Callum to talk by pursing my lips onto his little arm and speaking so that he could feel the vibrations from my lips. He loved the sensation and would laugh and try to copy me. Over 12 months of repeatedly talking on Rory's arm, he gradually learned to mimic my lip movements and make the right sounds for speech.

Help is always at hand

Some of the other medical professionals who may be involved in your child's therapy include:

- Audiologists, who assess hearing difficulties and advise on devices that can improve your child's hearing, such as hearing aids
- Educational psychologists, who assess and advise on children's learning and behaviour
- Neurologists, who are doctors specialising in the brain and nervous system
- Ophthalmologists, who are doctors specialising in the eye and vision problems
- Orthoptists, who assess vision problems and abnormal eye movements and demonstrate eye exercises, eye patching and other treatments for vision problems
- Paediatricians, who are doctors specialising in the care of children
- Psychologists, who assess emotional and behavioural issues and provide counselling.

I cannot emphasise enough how significant is the role that medical professionals play in supporting a child in Callum's situation. Health professionals are able to provide the help and resources that you need, quickly and easily. Recognise that people will readily help someone they like

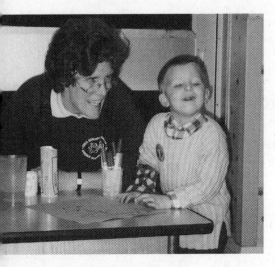

Ruth McAlister and Callum at the Child Development Centre, Airedale Hospital.

and will often put themselves out for those who appreciate their efforts; it's human nature. When your GP, physio, paediatric doctor or psychiatrist feels appreciated and you share a good rapport, the services and support seem to flow more readily.

In times of stress (and let's face it, even with healthy children that can be a large percentage of the time), we need to remember to remain civil and considerate. Most medical professionals choose a medical career because they want to help people in need. They tend to be very caring and generous people by nature, willing to do whatever it takes to make a difference. They have studied for many years in their dedication to helping others.

One of the problems I have encountered over the years is a habit that some medical professionals have of discussing a condition in language the average person doesn't understand. This often occurs because they have forgotten that parents are bewildered by all the medical

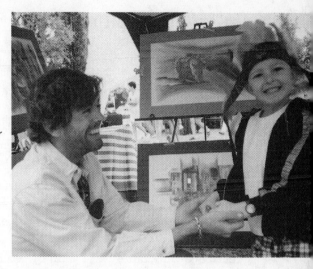

Life is full of colour

terminology relating to their child's condition. This some-times makes communication confusing. My advice is:

> If you don't understand what a doctor or therapist is telling you, ask them to explain it to you in straightforward language until you do.

This can make an enormous difference to how you relate to doctors and other medical personnel caring for your child. If you ever feel that you have a poor relationship with a medical professional or other therapist, find another doctor, or ask for support from someone with whom you communicate well. It is, after all, a team effort.

I cannot express enough thanks to Rory's team, who have diligently supported us both in the United Kingdom and Australia. Their help and advice have been invaluable.

Eating for a healthy body

> Your body is the temple of your soul.
> Keep looking after the walls of your temple
> so that those who pass by can admire the
> precious content.

Before you begin on any dietary or exercise program, or change your child's diet in any way, it is always wise to consult your doctor. Many children with cerebral palsy experience difficulties with eating, swallowing, digesting and processing food. Your doctor can advise on the best diet to suit your child's condition.

To function efficiently, our bodies need the right balance of food and water. If we are nourished with essential nutrients, oxygen, minerals and plenty of water, then our organs function efficiently and we have plenty of energy to get through the day. It is helpful to think of your body as being like a top-of-the-range Ferrari. If you put poor-quality fuel into your system or forget to top up your water supply, it may not be able to perform to maximum capacity. In fact, most high-performance cars are so finely tuned that they would simply break down if they were treated as poorly as many people treat their body. I know I made many mistakes myself.

If we abuse our system by eating the wrong foods, overeating or drinking too much alcohol, it can impact upon the rest of our body, leading to poor waste removal and illness. Many illnesses are related to poor eating habits

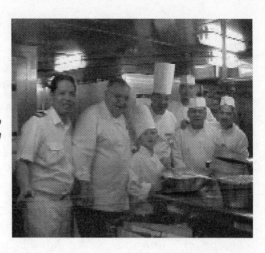

*Rory cooking up
a storm*

and inefficient waste removal because the liver, kidneys, bowel, blood and lymph systems are overloaded with toxins and impurities. Is it any wonder that we often feel lethargic and overweight?

Due to Callum's weak constitution and underdeveloped peristalsis (constriction and dilation of intestinal muscles to aid digestion) as a baby and later as a young boy, I always had to make sure he had a balanced diet which included lots of fruit and fibre. I would even supplement his normal school dinners and make sure he had fruit and high-fibre meals when we visited friends, otherwise he would suffer from constipation and terrible pain. I always knew when he was becoming more constipated, because his usually large appetite would diminish to hardly anything at all. The liquid laxative prescribed by the doctors would work wonders when he was suffering.

Food was a very touchy subject in my family. As mentioned before, both Mum and my sister are passionate and clever cooks. They were horrified that Callum could be so misinformed as to believe that his mother was a brilliant cook from the sound of a microwave 'dinging' and my offering five guests five different meals: Italian, Chinese, Mexican, Indian or Greek, at six-minute intervals! The choice was never-ending. And then of course there was my extensive supply of frozen Sara Lee cakes for dessert. As a reluctant chef, the microwave meal was my saviour.

Rory recently met Anthony Robbins at his 'Unleash the Power Within' seminar in Sydney, and he was invited to stay and enjoy the health section of the seminar, where we were shown footage of blood samples taken from a man on the morning before he was to undergo heart surgery and some days previously. His blood sample taken on the morning of the operation was full of yellow viscous fat – it was disgusting. His doctors were quite shocked by this blood sample, as his previous blood test was much clearer. They asked him what he had eaten the night before, and sheepishly he admitted that he had tucked into a popular fast-food chain hamburger, vanilla thick shake and fries.

We all make mistakes, and
no parent is perfect.

Rory and I looked at each other in horror, because during the meal break at 8 pm the previous day (an 8 pm 'lunchbreak' is the norm at Anthony Robbins's seminars – none of the participants want to leave, as they are glued to their seats with interest), Rory and I had raced out of the convention centre to grab that exact same meal. Rory exclaimed in dismay that I had been a bad mother for allowing him to eat his favourite meal! The visual impact of seeing this film was life-changing for us.

In addition, Dr William E. Ellis told us about studies demonstrating that malabsorption of calcium from cows' milk is harmful to humans. The mucus formed on the stomach lining when milk is consumed prevents the absorption of essential nutrients and it also neutralises the stomach acids that are needed to digest food. Over the years I had insisted that Rory drink double quotas of milk to 'help' with his bone development!

As a result of attending this seminar, Rory and I have become macrobiotic eaters – that is, we eat organic fruit, vegetables and eggs, as well as fish. We have also replaced cows' milk with rice milk, and we gain our calcium from broccoli.

> Nothing will benefit human health and increase chances of survival of life on Earth as much as the evolution to a vegetarian diet.
> ALBERT EINSTEIN

I gave Rory a big hug, and asked for his forgiveness. That evening I gave our freshly cooked chicken, milk and custard cartons to our wonderful neighbour, Sue, who was pleasantly surprised. Rory was disgusted and burst into tears, saying, 'Mummy, how can you possibly bear to poison our lovely neighbour?' To this day, Sue asks us whether we are still as passionate about being macrobiotic eaters, and indeed we are.

Now we prefer to eat five small meals a day, rather than the traditional three large meals a day. We have eliminated meat and dairy products from our diet and eat our carbohydrates (such as pasta, bread, potatoes and cereals), at different meal times to our protein foods (such as fish, eggs, nuts and beans). I believe that digestion is assisted when the stomach is able to process alkaline-based foods separately to acidic foods. Rory and I have also found that by drinking 12 glasses of water a day our energy levels have received an enormous boost. The method of 'water in, weight off' really works for us.

I have been fortunate to have never acquired the taste for alcohol, tea or coffee, so they have never been part of my diet. Chocolate and some cakes and sweets are my vice, but I have found that by eating healthily, my desire to eat unhealthy foods has diminished – okay, just a little. I'm human after all!

Up until this recent diet change I was of the opinion that a little bit of everything in moderation was fine, but this method doesn't work for a Ferrari. We cannot replace a Ferrari's petrol with gas or water. We have to put in just the right fuel for the Ferrari to perform at maximum capacity. So it is with our bodies.

With scientific research continually uncovering new findings about the human body and the relationship between diet, exercise, health and illness, we are becoming increasingly aware of the benefits of eating a healthy and balanced diet.

Alternative therapies

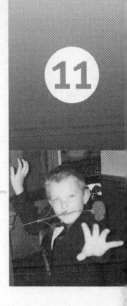

*The life given us by nature is short,
but the memory of a well-spent life
is eternal.*

Cicero

MANY PEOPLE ARE sceptical about the
benefits of 'alternative' and holistic therapies. Admittedly
many alternative therapies have not been scientifically
proven. However, an increasing number of medical
practitioners are embracing these alternative therapies.
In my experience, reflexology, massage, reiki, acupuncture, homeopathy and aromatherapy have a beneficial
effect on the body and the mind.

Throughout Rory's therapy program, and in my many
years of working in health spas, I have observed that
stimulating and caring for the body promotes positive

responses from the brain. A study by the University of Miami School of Medicine Touch Research Institute in 1997 demonstrated that autistic children given regular massage experienced improvements in their ability to relate to the world around them, including touch sensitivity, attention to sounds, classroom behaviour and relatedness to teachers.[10]

As you will see, I was willing to try all kinds of therapy as part of Rory's program. Some of these therapies may not be to your liking, but I recommend that in conjunction with the conventional medical treatment and therapies that your child receives, you keep an open mind about holistic and alternative therapies. The important thing is to trust your intuition about what works for you and your child. Following are brief descriptions of the alternative therapies that proved beneficial to Rory.

Yoga

The stretches and poses (known as 'asana') that are integral to this relaxing form of exercise can help to lengthen a child's muscles and tendons to relieve tightness and to ease problems of muscle tone. In yoga the spine is also stretched and realigned as a series of flexes and poses adjust the space between vertebrae, relieving pressure on radial nerves. By following a special series of yoga asana to stretch each muscle, a child with cerebral palsy can achieve greater coordination and a wider range of movements.

Massage

Giving massage and hugs to children is a great way to improve their energy and sense of wellbeing. If your child has cerebral palsy, their growth spurts will appear to set them back in their physiotherapy program because growth makes the muscles stiffen, hindering movement. Even if your children dance or play soccer, regular massaging helps by keeping the muscles warm, stimulated and relaxed, making movement easier.

I recommend massaging with a pre-mixed aromatherapy product that is grapeseed oil-based, but any body lotion will do, or use essential oils diluted in a carrier oil. Essential oils increase the vibration of the body. Scientists in Mexico have now linked essential oils to a possible cure for cancer. For centuries it has been understood that the skin absorbs essential oils. Not only do essential oils smell lovely, but they also have medicinal, antiseptic and healing properties.

Nearly 6000 years ago the Egyptian physician and god of medicine, Imhotep, used essential oils for massage therapy. In Ancient Greece, Hippocrates used aromatic fumigation to rid Athens of the Plague. Even in biblical times, essential oils were highly valued. The three wise kings are said to have brought gifts of frankincense oil, myrrh essential oil and 'gold', which is believed to be an alternative name used for the essential oil sandalwood, because of its wondrous properties.

Scientists now know that the human body, which is just another form of vibrating energy, vibrates at 70 to 90 MHz when in good health. Someone with flu or who consumes a lot of coffee vibrates at 62 MHz, while someone with cancer has an even lower vibration at 42 MHz. The essential oils actually increase the body's vibration. Research is now being carried out to establish how essential oils can be used in the treatment of cancer.

Always be sure to consult with a medical practitioner before using essential oils, as some essential oils may irritate the skin or be contraindicated for some medical conditions.

For some time, health practitioners have been aware of the benefits of massage and essential oils in pain relief. On several occasions I was employed by the Bradford Royal Infirmary to teach their McMillan cancer nurses massage with essential oils so that they could apply these techniques to their patients for pain relief.

I have always bathed Rory in essential oil baths. Six drops of pure essential oil is enough in a full bath. One of my clients had all his skin burnt off his feet after putting out a fire with his boots. Doctors placed dry bandages on his feet, but each day my client took it upon himself to bathe his feet in lavender essential oil. To the doctors' delight and amazement his feet healed and showed very little scarring within weeks rather than the months anticipated. The results speak for themselves.

Naturopathy
Naturopathy is like a 'health care system'. It uses only natural ingredients and disciplines. Treatment is varied and can include fasting, hydrotherapy, exercise and relaxation techniques.

Hippocrates, the Greek father of naturopathic medicine, embraced multi-disciplinary treatments and many natural ingredients. Naturopathy is a philosophy for life rather than a set of inflexible principles. Naturopaths aim to prevent and treat disease by detailed diagnosis and a wide array of treatments that must be integrated into a person's lifestyle if they are to work effectively in the long term.

Western herbalism

Western herbalism uses the curative qualities of plants to keep people healthy and balanced. It is an ancient art of healing and can ease a variety of ailments.

Herbs have been used in medicines for thousands of years. Herbalism forms part of the western heritage and it is equally important in Africa, India and China. Like most holistic practitioners, herbalists believe that we all possess healing energy within us. They call it the 'vital force'. This vital force works constantly to maintain our physical, mental and emotional health.

Reflexology

The ancient art of applying gentle pressure to certain points on the feet to relieve congestion and blockages in corresponding parts of the body is known as 'reflexology'. It was first used by the early Indian, Egyptian and Chinese cultures. Today reflexology is used to unblock congested energy points in the body caused by stress, illness or injury. Reflexologists believe that every part of the body has a corresponding point on the feet.

When I began to study reflexology I was just a few weeks pregnant. During one session of the course we had the opportunity to diagnose another student's condition. My fellow student, an experienced masseuse, was able to diagnose my pregnancy using reflexology, and I was equally surprised to be able to detect each of her problems that she had indicated on a sheet of paper hidden from me until the analysis was complete. I was most impressed, and consequently became quite fascinated by reflexology and all its health benefits. It is a very relaxing form of therapy.

Let me tell you a story. Before Rory was born, when his cousin Amber was only 18 months old, my sister Nichola had been very concerned about Amber's hearing and apparent earaches. As an experiment I decided to use one of the methods I was learning in the reflexology course, which involved massaging her feet and applying pressure to her second toe to stimulate pain relief for her ears. She had been to the doctor several times, and even though the doctor had examined her ears and found nothing, my sister was sure that Amber had a blockage in her ear canal. Boy oh boy, was her intuition right! Within the first five minutes of applying pressure, Amber began to whimper, then a volcanic rush of golden lava-like wax started to ooze from her ear. Nichola and I wanted to retch; it was like watching a sci-fi movie. The reflexology had saved the day. Amber was admitted to hospital for grommets to be inserted to ease her earaches and prevent further blockages. Subsequently Amber regained her *joie de vivre*, and her communication skills developed really quickly.

Reiki

Another form of massage spiritually linked to unblocking energy is reiki. It involves the transference of energy through the therapist to the client. I took Rory to a holistic healer who performed reiki massage after the doctors had suggested to me that he might never walk. The healer assured me that with plenty of daily massage and heat, Rory would learn to walk. His reassurance kept me hopeful

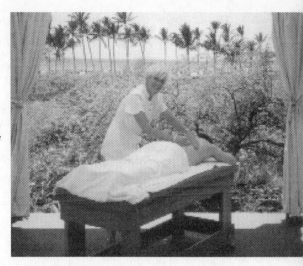

*Shelley performing
Reiki in Hawaii*

at a time when I was still very unsure of alternative therapies. I became a 'master' of reiki and I feel that my knowledge has certainly aided Rory's development, as well as helped many of my clients from around the world.

Homeopathy

Homeopathy is the use of plant, mineral or animal extracts diluted to very minute doses to stimulate the body's ability to heal itself. It first gained recognition in the nineteenth century after extensive research by the German pioneer, physician and chemist Samuel Hahn Mann, but it originates from the fifth century BC when Greek physician Hippocrates first introduced homeopathic remedies to the world. Homeopathy can help cure simple ailments like colds and stomach upsets, and more serious conditions like fibrosis and psoriasis. It is based on the belief that each person is different and individuals should be treated accordingly.

Homeopathy works on the principle that 'like should be treated with like', meaning that if the diluted extract used as a homeopathic remedy were present in a massive dose it would produce effects similar to the disease being treated. The aim is to use natural extracts to work in harmony with the immune system to treat the cause rather than just the symptoms of a particular condition. For example, hepar sulphate (hepar sulphurise calcaneum) in the form of a tiny tablet is a favoured homeopathic remedy for acne. It is said to work by stimulating the body to stop overproducing the hormones that cause adolescent acne. It is prepared from burning the white interior of oyster shells with pure flowers of sulphur. The tablets are minute and are made from natural substances, unlike many of the chemically produced tablets manufactured by pharmaceutical companies.

I have used a host of homeopathy remedies at home for Rory and me, including arnica for cuts and bruises; argent nit for sugar cravings, headache, colic and tummy upset; belladonna for Rory's swollen joints and air sickness; and calcium carbonate for weight loss, cold hands and toothache. Homeopaths can diagnose and recommend homeopathic remedies specific to your symptoms.

Din Y San

The Din Y San machine was invented in China to gauge the body's resistance using homeopathic substances. It checks for food intolerances, vitamin and mineral deficiencies and chemical resistances. In just one hour, approximately 88 tests can be conducted in a non-invasive fashion. The Din Y San machine is able to quickly determine why someone is feeling tired, or why children may be hyperactive or suffer from such ailments as eczema. It can also check acupuncture points to reveal any imbalances in the liver, spleen, lungs, heart and other organs.

It was a friend who suggested that I consult with a Chinese medicine man after expressing my concerns that my doctor wanted to prescribe to me Prozac, an anti-depressant, because I was feeling tired and weepy. I just knew that I wasn't suffering from depression – I had come to terms with my divorce, work was going well and Rory was healthy and happy. During the 88 tests, the Din Y San indicator rose right off the scale at the aspartame measure. 'What is aspartame?' I asked. The operator told me that aspartame is an artificial sweetener 150 to 200 times sweeter than sugar, which is used as a low-calorie substitute for sugar in diet drinks, tinned food and microwave meals. He needn't have said anything more ... I was drinking ten cans of diet drink per day and living on at least one to two microwave meals per day. I had effectively poisoned myself!

The rest of the test showed that I was fine apart from a deficiency of some B-complex vitamins. I immediately stopped consuming diet drinks and eating microwave meals. Within one week I started to feel great once again. A month later I went back for a second check-up and was given the all clear.

I was sure that many people were being medicated for their symptoms rather than the cause of their symptoms being treated, so I decided that my staff and I would train on these machines. I purchased one for each spa. We helped thousands of people, from children with eczema to women with weight and fatigue problems. It was amazing each time to discover that they had an imbalance of a particular mineral or nutrient. Frequently our clients would take their results to their medical practitioner who had been unable to pinpoint the cause of their malady.

Since that time I have never drunk diet drinks again, although I must admit I do have microwave dinners! But I also have a Din Y San check-up once every six months to verify that all is well.

Acupuncture

Acupuncture is a traditional Chinese medical technique that uses needles to stimulate energy points in the body, and which aims to restore the body's balance, improve overall wellbeing and alleviate pain. Stone acupuncture needles dating back from as far as the Neolithic period (2500 BC) have been found in tombs in Mongolia.

Acupuncture literally means 'needle piercing'. Very fine needles are inserted into the skin to stimulate specific points called acupoints in order to balance the movement of energy in the body. Traditional Chinese philosophy states that the energy of the body, or 'Chi', needs to flow freely through the body's 14 meridians or pathways. Chi is said to consist of opposite female and male qualities known as Yin and Yang, which need to be balanced in order to enjoy good physical, emotional and spiritual health. The body's energy flow can be unbalanced by stress, poor nutrition and any number of physical, emotional or spiritual factors.

Both Rory and I have had acupuncture treatments, Rory to help reduce the swelling and pain in his knees and to rebalance his energy levels, and me to de-stress, as a form of pain relief after serious whiplash, and to help regain good posture. Neither Rory nor I enjoy needles, yet I find acupuncture surprisingly soothing ... although I do admit to keeping my eyes closed during treatment!

LaStone® Therapy

LaStone therapy is a form of massage therapy that uses alternating hot and chilled stones applied to the body to bring about healing and balance to physical, mental and emotional energy. It is based on the traditional healing practices of the native Americans. Memories and emotions can be released by this energising therapy, and some people enter quite a deep meditative state during treatment. Rory has never quite been able to explain how LaStone therapy helps him, other than to say that it makes him feel great and very relaxed. He loves the feel, smell and touch of the massage and the stones. I have certainly found it to be a very relaxing and calming therapy.

Crystal therapy

Crystals are used today in many modern technologies, particularly in electronics and in the optical industry. Crystal particles form into a wide variety of geometrical shapes, depending on the internal arrangement of atoms and molecules. They are formed by the solidification of chemicals. Crystals are said to channel energy, carrying vibrations that resonate with the chakras to boost the body's energy flow. They are also said to assist with emotional healing and in boosting the immune system. The human body constantly vibrates at a particular frequency. If a person is ill or has an imbalance of some sort, their body resonates at a low frequency, but if they are in good health, it resonates at a high frequency. Crystals and essential oils assist by rebalancing the frequency of the body's vibrations to the natural level.

Every now and then Rory instinctively walks around the house holding a crystal or puts one under his pillow. He says he does this when he experiences a sudden urge to have a crystal close by. He believes that crystals help to rebalance him.

We all need our energy tanks replenished from time to time, and it is at these times that I give Rory big hugs and kisses as a double insurance that he feels energised and well.

Feng shui

The Chinese art of feng shui involves following particular rules regarding architecture and the position of objects for health, wealth and happiness. A feng shui practitioner aims to balance the Yin and Yang of your physical surroundings to create harmony, wellbeing and success. It makes sense to me that if we are simply vibrating energy matter like everything else in the universe, we will be affected by the other energy forces that apply to the rest of the planet, such as gravity, the tides, the moon, and the ebb and flow of energy from the people around us.

My friend Suzanne introduced me to the art of feng shui over 12 years ago. I was fascinated to discover that my natural decorating style corresponded very closely to the principals of feng shui. My spas, with their mirrors, water features and colours, and the location of the desks, beds and so on, were all in harmony with the Chinese principals of balance and energy flow for abundance and wellbeing. Through my passion for style and wellbeing, I have been able to develop expertise in this field, working with architects, on TV lifestyle programs and applying my knowledge to benefit others.

Electromagnetic frequency balancing (EMF)

EMF involves the releasing of negative vibrations that are attached to your outer aura or magnetic field. After undergoing a great deal of personal development and adopting a new healthy eating regime, I decided while on holiday in the beautiful town of Broome, Western Australia, to visit Chinatown. There I was directed to a herbalist and healer's shop, where the healer was passionate about EMF treatments. I decided to carry out my own market research by booking myself in for a treatment.

I was escorted into a highly decorated room with pictures of saints, swags of brightly coloured silks, candles, crystals and the scent of burning incense. After requesting that the universe direct the healer to find my healing colour, I was covered with a blue silk, and a host of crystals were placed around my body and on my chakra points. The healer used stones, crystals and colours to increase my sense of wellbeing. The healer perceptively picked up from my energies or vibrations that I needed to be careful to replenish my reserves of love and energy after giving to others.

EMF treatments clear the body's vibrations, helping you to feel very calm and relaxed. That has certainly been my experience of EMF. Some people find it to be an emotional but cathartic experience.

Trust your intuition

Always trust your gut feelings when choosing a therapy, but keep an open mind to the various options available to you, whether they have been scientifically proven or not. Put together a program that works for you and your child by increasing your sense of health and wellbeing.

> If you have a strong intuitive feeling, listen to it.

My willingness to try alternative therapies even extended to taking Rory to the Bahamas after hearing about a special centre where groups of people are invited to swim with dolphins. These wonderful creatures are said to have special sensory acquity, particularly with sick and disabled people. I had heard amazing reports of some people's 'life-changing experiences', so I wanted Rory to have the opportunity to be touched by the dolphins.

A trainer guides the dolphins to swim up to people who are standing in the water. Because Rory was only four years old, I was advised to hold him in front of me and stay still as the dolphins made their approach. The dolphins headed straight for Rory, nudging him and allowing him to stroke their rubbery bodies. He got their full attention and laughed and giggled. It was a wonderfully uplifting experience for him.

I believe that there are energies in the universe that we don't fully comprehend, and I challenge you as parents to allow magic into your lives and be willing to accept the benefits of alternative therapies without always needing to understand precisely how they work.

Physical closeness

Hugs and kisses have always played a big part in our family. We are passionate and demonstrative people. Physical closeness feels good, and giving or receiving a hug – no matter what your age, the time of day or where you are – is uplifting. However, some people abuse this gift, and sadly we often hear about children being physically abused by their family, friends or neighbours. These incidents leave their mark and it can take a long time for the victim to heal. Sometimes the trauma is carried over to the next generation.

I have discovered over the years that the best way to approach other adults is to mirror their behaviour. Some people need more space and are less touchy-feely than others. They would feel uncomfortable if someone they had only just met embraced them. Other people feel quite comfortable about hugging someone they have just met. The key is to be you and learn to read other people's body language to accurately gauge what they are comfortable with.

Rory and I have a wonderful bond. We laugh and joke when he sits on my knee and I say, 'Gee, what happened to my baby? You're massive now.' He loves it when I lift him into my arms when we are in the water (the only

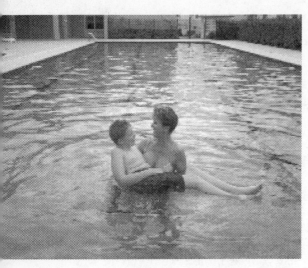

Shelley and Rory at home in Sydney

place I can lift him these days) as if he was a baby in my arms. These little precious moments just reaffirm our love and connection. I hope we never lose this bond.

Appendix

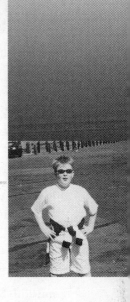

There is no passion to be found in playing small – in settling for a life that is less than what you are capable of living.

Nelson Mandela

2B1 Sanctuary

Until we are personally affected by suffering, we may not realise the significance of the assistance given by so many hospitals and charitable organisations. It is wonderful to know that there are so many dedicated people, from physiotherapists, nurses and doctors, to surgeons, eye specialists, psychologists and countless other medical professionals, who work tirelessly to improve the quality of life of the children and families in their care.

These hospitals are a sanctuary for many children suffering from birth or growth defects, or being treated for injuries caused by child abuse. They can seem shocking places to anyone who has never witnessed suffering on such a scale before. Thankfully there are many hospitals and charities making a difference.

Dr Ward, Rory's paediatrician in England, suggested that if I really wanted to show my gratitude to her team in a practical way, raising money for more intensive care units would be ideal. In 1993 I organised the inaugural Beautiful Ball to raise much-needed funds for children's intensive care units. It seemed logical to me for friends and contacts to enjoy a great party while raising funds for a worthwhile cause.

The inaugural Beautiful Ball was so successful that many guests booked their tickets for the following year as they left. The Beautiful Ball is now an annual event, has raised thousands of pounds, and has now crossed continents to Australia.

There are also many charities that help with funding breaks for parents, children's holiday camps, and who can provide such assistance as organising a new washing machine if yours breaks down. I made use of this help when I was desperate after my marriage breakdown and before I was receiving income support.

One of the best ways to help is to find a charity that is significant to you in some way. Whether it involves raising funds or helping in the community or counselling others, participating in this way transforms you from a victim and recipient to an activist caring for others' wellbeing.

As a committee member of several charities, and

having raised Rory with all the difficulties that that entailed and achieving some amazing results, it became evident to me that many charitable organisations are working towards the same goal – to raise the community's consciousness about positive parenting skills and to empower children to reach their potential. As a result, these charities have now teamed together to work with corporations and the community at large. I have registered a charity called the 2B1 Foundation and with the help of Natalie Simon have put together a business plan that we are hoping will be taken under the wing of some magnanimous donors who are keen to help children and parents from all corners of the world. I have my fingers crossed that this ambitious project will come to fruition.

Our challenge is to open a health sanctuary in Australia for children and parents, called 2B1 Sanctuary. This will be modelled on the Sol Kurzner 'Sun City' complex in South Africa, with the important difference being that the 2B1 Sanctuary will be run by a charitable organisation. The sanctuary will consist of magnificent hotels, gardens, water pools and a spiritually uplifting haven where love, healing, personal development, values and beliefs can be realigned, and where bigger dreams can be envisaged.

The sanctuary will offer physiotherapy, counselling, yoga, reiki, acupuncture, meditation, life-coaching for children and parents, Chinese medicine, homeopathy, allergy testing, crystal therapy, writing classes, drama and music studios, colour therapy rooms, flotation tanks, beauty spas and massage therapy. There will also be an auditorium where stars and mentors such as Deepak Chopra, Brian Tracy and Anthony Robbins will be invited to share their wisdom with a large audience comprising of school groups, hospital staff, corporate businesses, parents, volunteers, healers and children from around the world staying at the sanctuary. This will be partially financed by a five-star hotel that will accommodate the children and parents visiting the sanctuary, and will also be open to anyone else who is willing to pay for the enjoyment of the luxury complex. The presence of celebrities or leaders, if they wish to be acknowledged, will be a motivation to the children and others that dreams can come true.

Children who are guests at the sanctuary will be able to enjoy the full range of therapies and services available, to help them to focus on being the best they can be and have the confidence to follow their dreams. Parents will have the opportunity to develop the life skills to bring out the best in themselves and their children.

We intend to continue the funding of the 2B1 Sanctuary through donations, sales in the hotel, TV programs, book sales, and through our functions and parties. We hope that many generous doctors, psychologists, life coaches, nurses and specialists will be willing to contribute their skills by working with us for a couple of weeks at a time on secondment.

Please write to us in 100 words or less what '2B1' means to you, and you may be the first lucky parent, child, nurse, therapist or healer to be invited to the opening of the 2B1 Sanctuary and have your ideas presented on our website.

If you would like to work at the sanctuary or help raise funds, please contact us at our website:

www.shelleysykes.com/charities

Charitable organisations

Whatever charity you choose to support, someone's life will be better for it. I truly believe that the more you give in life the more you receive. Donate from your heart, and remember, it is just as rewarding to give as to receive.

Asthma Australia
National Office
Level 3, 63 Stead Street
South Melbourne VIC 3205
Tel: 03 9696 7861
Fax: 03 9696 7393
Email: national@asthma.org.au
<http://www.asthmaaustralia.org.au>

Australian Cerebral Palsy Association
PO Box 237
Woodville SA 5011
Tel: 08 8347 4588
<http://www.acpa-inc.org.au>

Giant Steps
Giant Steps is a charity for children with autism and learning/behavioural difficulties.

PO Box 2091
Gladesville NSW 1675
Tel: 02 9879 4971
Email: sandy.durrant@giantsteps.net.au
<http://www.giantsteps.net.au>

The House With No Steps
Head Office
49 Blackbutts Road
Belrose NSW 2085
Tel: 02 9451 1511
<http://www.hwns.com.au>

Formerly The Wheelchair and Disabled Association of
Australia, the mission of The House With No Steps is to
enhance the lives of people with disabilities and to make
the most of people's abilities through quality support
services such as employment services, residential support,
and recreation programs.

The Lord's Taverners Australia
The Lord's Taverners Australia is an organisation that
gives the young, the disadvantaged and the disabled a
sporting chance.

16 Daisy Street
Croydon Park NSW 2133
Tel: 02 9744 9255
Email: lordstavnsw@optusnet.com.au

Magic Moments Foundation Limited
The Magic Moments Foundation Australia is a non-profit
organisation formed to assist the personal development of
children who have not had the best start in life and other
people who are often forgotten by society – the homeless,
elderly, needy families, and anyone else needing a
'helping hand'. Magic Moments is linked to the Anthony
Robbins Foundation, Discovery Camp and Basket Brigade.

PO Box 276
St Leonards NSW 1590
Tel: 02 9966 4472
Fax: 02 9966 4474
<http://www.magicmoments.org.au>

The Spastic Centre

The Spastic Centre is the major provider of services to people with cerebral palsy of all ages in New South Wales. The Centre's mission is to support people with cerebral palsy, and their families. Services include: technology, therapy, conductive education, equipment loan, Hart Walker program, employment, respite care, information, family support, accommodation, aquatic programs, rural outreach, recreation. The Spastic Centre website features an extensive range of information for people with cerebral palsy, their families, students and other service providers: <http://www.thespasticcentre.org.au>

Head Office: 189 Allambie Road
Allambie Heights NSW 2100
(PO Box 184
Brookvale NSW 2100)
Tel: 02 9451 9022
Fax: 02 9451 4877
Email: scnsw@tscnsw.org.au
Ryde Centre
PO Box 333
Ryde NSW 1680
Tel: 02 9809 7055

TLC for Kids Inc.

This association raises money for children's activities, outings and equipment, especially for those children who don't live with their parents or whose families don't have adequate finances.

PO Box 1044
Niddrie VIC 3042
Tel: 03 98638311
<http://www.tlcforkids.org.au>

Other organisations

Basket Brigade

Basket Brigade is the annual Christmas activity of the Magic Moments Foundation, founded in 1995. There are currently nine Basket Brigades throughout Australia, each organising the collection of food, gifts, books, new clothes, toys, toiletries, and cash to purchase the food to make up the baskets.

The Basket Brigade delivers anonymously to people in need. A card is left inside the box, which says 'this basket is from someone who cares for you. All that we ask is that you take care of yourself well enough to be able to do this for someone else some day'.

We invite you to join us as a volunteer or coordinator to work in your own community to make a difference.

Anthony Robbins Foundation

The Anthony Robbins Youth leadership 'Discovery Camp' and mentoring program are run by committed volunteers whose goal is to create the opportunity for young people to set their own standards for their future.

Maureen Kilkenny
Executive Director
Anthony Robbins Foundation
9888 Carroll Centre Road
Suite 112
San Diego CA 92126
Tel: 800 554 0619 or
    800 535 6295
Email: maureenk@tonyrobbins.com
<http://www.basketbrigade.org/cig/index.ph>

BaySports Association

The BaySports Association was set up to operate as an independent not-for-profit organisation. Its aim is to foster and promote sport and recreation for small clubs in Canada Bay so that the club organiser's time and energy can be fully focused on training the children and developing their clubs.

Tel: 02 9713 4322
4 William Street
Five Dock NSW

Centrelink

Centrelink is the government agency that delivers a range of services to the Australian community. Centrelink can assist if you are: ill, injured or have a disability; caring for someone who is aged, ill or disabled; a parent or guardian; looking for work; recently separated or divorced; in crisis or requiring special help; needing help after someone has died;

planning for or needing help after retirement; recently
settled in Australia; planning to study or undertake training;
self-employed or responsible for a farm.
Tel: Customer Relations: FreeCALL™ 1800 050 004
    Disability, Sickness and Carers: 13 2717
    Multilingual Call: 13 1202
http://www.centrelink.gov.au

Great4Life Pty Ltd
The Ultimate Lifestyle and Fitness Results
Level 29 Chifley Tower
Sydney NSW 2000
Tel: 02 9251 6680
<http://www.great4life.com>

Sydney Children's Hospital
High Street
Randwick NSW 2031
Tel: 02 9382 1111

Alternative therapy organisations

Association of Remedial Masseurs
Suite 3/120 Blaxland Rd
Ryde NSW 2112
(PO Box 440
Ryde NSW 1680)
Tel: 02 9807 4769

Association of Traditional Medicine Society Ltd
Tel: 02 9809 6800

Australian Acupuncture and Chinese Medicine Association
National Administration & Practitioner Referrals
Suite 5/28 Gladstone Road
Highgate Hill QLD 4101
Tel: 1300 725 334

Australian Association of Yoga in Daily Life
102 Booth Street
Annandale NSW 2038
Tel: 02 9518 7788

Australian Homeopathic Association
Tel: 08 8346 3961

International Federation of Aromatherapists Inc.
Tel: 03 9850 9254

Reflexology Association of Australia
Tel: 0500 502 250

Further reading

Canfield, J. and Hansen, M.V. 1996, *Chicken Soup for the Soul*, Health Communications, Inc., Florida.

Carnegie, D. 1985 *How to Stop Worrying and Start Living*, Pocket Books, New York.

Carnegie, D. 1990, *How to Win Friends and Influence People*, Pocket Books, New York.

Coelho, P. 1985, *The Alchemist*, Harper, San Francisco.

Fitzgerald, T. 2002, *Start Me Up*, Simon and Schuster, Sydney.

Gawain, S. 1988, *Living in the Light: A Guide to Personal and Planetary Transformation*, New World Library, Novato, CA.

Gray, Dr J. 2000, *How to Get What You Want and Want What You Have*, HarperCollins, New York.

Harrold, F. 2002, *Be Your Own Life Coach*, Hodder & Stoughton, London.

Hill, N. 1990, *Think and Grow Rich*, Fawcett Books, New York.

Kiyosaki, R. 2000, *Rich Dad Poor Dad*, Warner Books, New York.

Koran, A. 1988, *Bring out the Magic in Your Mind*, HarperCollins, New York.

McGinnes, A.L., 1993, *The Power of Optimism*, HarperCollins, New York.

McGrath, J. 2000, *You Don't Have to Be Born Brilliant*, Hodder Headline, Sydney.

Matthews, A. 1990, *Being Happy*, Media Masters, Sydney.

Matthews, A. 1997, *Follow Your Heart*, Seashell Books, Trinity Beach.

Redfield, J. 1997, *The Celestine Prophecy*, Warner Books, New York.

Robbins, A. 1993, *Awaken the Giant Within*, Fireside, New York.

Tracy, B. 1989, *The Psychology of Success: Ten Universal Principles for Personal Empowerment/Audio Cassettes*, Nightingale-Conant Corporation, Niles, IL.

Waitley, Dr D. 1983, *The Winner's Edge: The Critical Attitude of Success*, Berkley Books, New York.

Walsch, N. 1991, *Conversations with God: An Uncommon Dialogue*, Penguin Putnam, New York.

Young-Sowers, M.L. 1984, *Agartha*, Stillpoint, Walpole, NH.

Notes

Chapter 1

1 Spastic Centre of New South Wales, 2001, *The Children's Services Newsletter*, Metropolitan North and East Region, Issue 2, August 2001.

2 Murdoch Children's Research Institute, 2003, Melbourne, viewed 20 June 2003, <http://murdoch.rch.unimelb.edu.au/pages/child_health /cerebral_palsy.html>

3 Australia, Senate 2001, *Matters of Public Interest*, Allison, Sen. Lyn, viewed 20 June 2003, <http://wipi.aph.gov.au/search/>

Chapter 9

4 Australian Bureau of Statistics, *Children, Australia: A Social Report*, 1999, viewed 9 April 2003, <http://www.abs.gov.au/ausstats/>

5 Australian Bureau of Statistics, 2001, *Births Australia 2000*, Cat 3301.0, Canberra, ABS.

6 Australian Institute of Criminology, 2003, Media release, viewed 13 May 2003, <www.aic.gov.au/media/>

7 U.S. Bureau of the Census, 1998, Washington, D.C., 'Co-resident Grandparents and Their Grandchildren:

Grandparent Maintained Families', *Population Division Working Paper No. 26*, viewed 13 May 2003, <http://landview.census.gov/population/www/document ation/twps0026.html>

8 UNICEF Statistics, 'Fertility and Contraceptive Use', viewed 20 June 2003, <http://www.childinfo.org/eddb/fertility/index.htm>

9 Australian Bureau of Statistics, *Year Book Australia 2002*, 'Centenary Article – Child Health Since Federation', viewed 8 May 2003, <http://www.abs.gov.au/>

Chapter 11

10 Field, T., Lasko, D., Mundy, P., Henteleff, T., Talpins, S., & Dowling, M. 1997, 'Autistic Children's Attentiveness and Responsivity Improve After Touch Therapy, *Journal of Autism & Developmental Disorders, 27*, 333–338, , viewed 1 May 2003, <http://www.miami.edu/touch-research/index.html>

Babies! A Parent's Guide to Enjoying Baby's First Year

Dr Christopher Green

The arrival of a baby is one of the most memorable events in a parent's life. It is an exciting time, yet many mums and dads feel overwhelmed and are not sure what to do.

This second edition of *Babies!* is packed with practical, commonsense, up-to-date advice that will give every parent the confidence to enjoy their child's first year.

Dr Christopher Green is Australia's best-known parenting author. For more than 20 years he has helped parents with advice on babies, toddlers and young children, and his humorous, no-nonsense approach has preserved the sanity of many mums and dads. A paediatrician and honorary consultant to the Children's Hospital, Westmead, Sydney, Dr Green's legendary sleep technique is now used worldwide.

ISBN 0 7318 1093 7
Paperback
328 pp
224 × 165 mm

So You're Going to be a Dad

Peter Downey

Finally, here is the first guide written especially for unsuspecting Australian males who know little or nothing about parenting but are keen to have a go. A book that explodes the myths – a tough, uncompromising, no-holds-barred, no beg-your-pardons look at fatherhood, from the sperm that started it all to the sleep deprivation you'll suffer as a consequence.

So You're Going to be a Dad is a wry and very funny book about the trials and joys of parenting. It also provides useful and practical advice about pregnancy, childbirth and baby care, and examines issues of vital importance. Complete with a glossary full of handy words you'll need to know and a lot more that you won't, plus the films to watch and the ones to avoid, and words of wisdom from real live fathers, *So You're Going to be a Dad* is without doubt one of the greatest parental education books ever written.

ISBN 0 7318 0464 3
Paperback
208 pp
222 × 162 mm

Everyone Can Win: How to Resolve Conflict

Helena Cornelius & Shoshana Faire

Have you ever slammed a door in rage? Have you ever been really hurt by something someone has said? Have you ever had a fight with your mother? Have you ever been angry when your pay rise was turned down?

Every day people find themselves in conflict, ranging from minor discomfort to serious confrontations. Generally when people think about conflict they believe that there are only three solutions: compromising, winning or losing. But now, *Everyone Can Win* provides a new way to look at winning so that opponents become partners.

Everyone Can Win shows how to recognise typical conflict behaviour patterns and how to avoid them. As well it teaches us how to understand the power dynamics in a relationship. Most importantly, however, it shows how improved communication can help us to better understand those with whom we find ourselves in conflict, and help them to understand us, in order to achieve a happy solution.

With its friendly advice, entertaining cartoons and proven techniques, *Everyone Can Win* is an inspirational sourcebook for all those who want to win – and who want everyone else to win, too.

ISBN 0 7318 0111 3
Paperback
192 pp
224 × 165 mm